Pediatric Allergy

Editor

DAVID R. STUKUS

IMMUNOLOGY AND ALLERGY CLINICS OF NORTH AMERICA

www.immunology.theclinics.com

Consulting Editor
STEPHEN A. TILLES

November 2019 • Volume 39 • Number 4

ELSEVIER

1600 John F. Kennedy Boulevard • Suite 1800 • Philadelphia, Pennsylvania, 19103-2899
http://www.theclinics.com

IMMUNOLOGY AND ALLERGY CLINICS OF NORTH AMERICA Volume 39, Number 4
November 2019 ISSN 0889-8561, ISBN-13: 978-0-323-68312-8

Editor: Katerina Heidhausen
Developmental Editor: Kristen Helm

Immunology and Allergy Clinics of North America (ISSN 0889–8561) is published quarterly by Elsevier Inc., 360 Park Avenue South, New York, NY 10010-1710. Months of issue are February, May, August, and November. Periodicals postage paid at New York, NY and additional mailing offices. Subscription prices are $341.00 per year for US individuals, $593.00 per year for US institutions, $100.00 per year for US students and residents, $423.00 per year for Canadian individuals, $220.00 per year for Canadian students, $753.00 per year for Canadian institutions, $447.00 per year for international individuals, $753.00 per year for international institutions, $220.00 per year for international students. To receive student/resident rate, orders must be accompanied by name of affiliated institution, date of term, and the *signature* of program/residency coordinator on institution letterhead. Orders will be billed at individual rate until proof of status is received. Foreign air speed delivery is included in all *Clinics* subscription prices. All prices are subject to change without notice. **POSTMASTER:** Send address changes to *Immunology and Allergy Clinics of North America*, Elsevier Health Sciences Division, Subscription Customer Service, 3251 Riverport Lane, Maryland Heights, MO 63043. **Customer Service: 1-800-654-2452 (U.S. and Canada); 314-447-8871 (outside U.S. and Canada). Fax: 314-447-8029. E-mail: journalscustomerservice-usa@elsevier.com (for print support); journalsonlinesupport-usa@elsevier.com (for online support).**

Reprints. For copies of 100 or more, of articles in this publication, please contact the Commercial Reprints Department, Elsevier Inc., 360 Park Avenue South, New York, New York 10010-1710. Tel. 212-633-3874, Fax: 212-633-3820, E-mail: reprints@elsevier.com.

Immunology and Allergy Clinics of North America is covered in MEDLINE/PubMed (Index Medicus), Current Contents/Life Sciences, Science Citation Index, ISI/BIOMED, Chemical Abstracts, and EMBASE/Excerpta Medica.

Printed in the United States of America.

Contributors

CONSULTING EDITOR

STEPHEN A. TILLES, MD
Senior Director, Medical Affairs, Aimmune Therapeutics, Brisbane, California, USA;
Clinical Professor of Medicine, University of Washington, Seattle, Washington, USA

EDITOR

DAVID R. STUKUS, MD
Associate Professor of Pediatrics, Division of Allergy and Immunology, Nationwide
Children's Hospital, The Ohio State University College of Medicine, Columbus, Ohio, USA

AUTHORS

ELISSA M. ABRAMS, MD
Department of Pediatrics, Section of Allergy and Clinical Immunology, University of
Manitoba, Winnipeg, Manitoba, Canada

NEHA T. AGNIHOTRI, MD
Fellow, Department of Medicine, Division of Allergy and Immunology, Northwestern
University Feinberg School of Medicine, Chicago, Illinois, USA

WILLIAM C. ANDERSON III, MD
Assistant Professor, Department of Pediatrics, Division of Allergy and Immunology,
Children's Hospital Colorado, University of Colorado School of Medicine, Aurora,
Colorado, USA

JACLYN BJELAC, MD
Cleveland Clinic Children's Hospital, Cleveland Clinic Pediatric Allergy, Cleveland,
Ohio, USA

EDMOND S. CHAN, MD
Department of Pediatrics, Division of Allergy and Immunology, University of British
Columbia, BC Children's Hospital, Vancouver, British Columbia, Canada

HEY J. CHONG, MD, PhD
Department of Pediatrics, UPMC Children's Hospital of Pittsburgh, Pittsburgh,
Pennsylvania, USA

HANNAH DUFFEY, MD
Department of Pediatrics, Division of Allergy and Immunology, Children's Hospital
Colorado, University of Colorado School of Medicine, Aurora, Colorado, USA

JUSTIN GREIWE, MD
Bernstein Allergy Group Inc, Division of Immunology/Allergy Section, Department of
Internal Medicine, The University of Cincinnati College of Medicine, Cincinnati, Ohio, USA

RUCHI S. GUPTA, MD, MPH
Professor of Pediatrics and Medicine, Institute for Public Health and Medicine, Northwestern University Feinberg School of Medicine, Ann & Lurie Children's Hospital of Chicago, Chicago, Illinois, USA

JENNIFER HEIMALL, MD
Division of Allergy and Immunology, Children's Hospital of Philadelphia, Philadelphia, Pennsylvania, USA

MONICA T. KRAFT, MD
Resident, Department of Pediatrics, Nationwide Children's Hospital, Columbus, Ohio, USA

DAWN K. LEI, MD
Fellow, Department of Medicine, Division of Allergy and Immunology, Northwestern University Feinberg School of Medicine, Chicago, Illinois, USA

SCOTT MAURER, MD
Department of Pediatrics, UPMC Children's Hospital of Pittsburgh, Pittsburgh, Pennsylvania, USA

IRENE J. MIKHAIL, MD
Assistant Professor, Division of Allergy and Immunology, Nationwide Children's Hospital, Columbus, Ohio, USA

SABRINA PALACIOS, MD
Assistant Professor, Department of Pediatrics, Division of Pulmonary Medicine, Nationwide Children's Hospital, The Ohio State University College of Medicine, Columbus, Ohio, USA

ANDREJ A. PETROV, MD
Section Chief of Allergy, Division of Pulmonary, Allergy and Critical Care Medicine, Associate Professor, Department of Medicine, University of Pittsburgh Medical Center, Pittsburgh, Pennsylvania, USA

BENJAMIN T. PRINCE, MD, MSCI
Assistant Professor, Department of Pediatrics, Division of Allergy and Immunology, Nationwide Children's Hospital, The Ohio State University College of Medicine, Columbus, Ohio, USA

REKHA RAVEENDRAN, MD
Assistant Professor of Internal Medicine, Division of Allergy/Immunology, Department of Otolaryngology, The Ohio State University Wexner Medical Center, OSU Eye and Ear Institute, Columbus, Ohio, USA

BRIAN SCHROER, MD
Director of Allergy and Immunology, Akron Children's Hospital, Akron, Ohio, USA

DAVID R. STUKUS, MD
Associate Professor of Pediatrics, Division of Allergy and Immunology, Nationwide Children's Hospital, The Ohio State University College of Medicine, Columbus, Ohio, USA

LISA ULRICH, MD
Assistant Professor, Department of Pediatrics, Division of Pulmonary Medicine, Nationwide Children's Hospital, The Ohio State University College of Medicine, Columbus, Ohio, USA

Contents

Thus far, the most effective strategy for the prevention of food allergy is early introduction of allergenic solids to at-risk infants. Early skin moisturization may have a role in food allergy prevention. There is insufficient evidence for hydrolyzed formula as a means of allergy prevention. Studies on vitamin D, omega 3, and probiotic supplementation; breastfeeding; early infant dietary diversity; and maternal peanut ingestion during pregnancy and breastfeeding are inconsistent.

A landmark study showed that early peanut introduction in high-risk infants, defined as infants with moderate to severe atopic dermatitis or egg allergy, reduced the risk of developing peanut allergy. Since this trial, many international societies have updated feeding guidelines to promote early introduction of peanut, usually around 6 months of age. Implementing these guidelines on a national and international level has been challenging. Furthermore, there is confusion if allergy testing is needed before peanut introduction in high-risk infants. Despite these challenges, the data are promising, that implantation of early introduction guidelines can reduce the burden of peanut allergy.

Current guidelines state that there is insufficient evidence to recommend testing siblings of food allergic children before introduction of potential allergic foods, but the topic continues to remain controversial. Although the proportion of siblings who are sensitized to a food without clinical reactivity is high in comparison to those with a true food allergy, there is still a known increased risk amongst siblings of children with food allergies that has led to much apprehension about management. The appropriateness of testing and further steps for management of sensitization in the absence of history of clinical reactivity should be discussed with parents.

Newborn screening for severe combined immunodeficiency has been implemented in all 50 states. This screening identifies newborns with T-cell lymphopenia. After an abnormal screening, additional testing is needed to determine if the child has severe combined immunodeficiency. Because screening programs vary, it is imperative for the clinical immunologist to understand how screening is done in their state and to prepare an effective assessment protocol for the management of these patients. Part of this assessment should include training and helping to ensure the effective delivery of this news to the family, a skill neither intuitive nor classically taught to immunologists.

Vocal cord dysfunction (VCD) is an upper airway disorder characterized by exaggerated and transient glottic constriction causing respiratory and laryngeal symptoms. Although the origin of VCD symptoms is in the upper airway, it is frequently misdiagnosed as asthma resulting in significant morbidity. VCD can coexist with asthma or mimic allergic conditions affecting the upper airway. VCD may be difficult to diagnose, because patients are intermittently symptomatic and VCD awareness in the medical community is underappreciated. Once VCD is diagnosed and treated, most patients report significant improvement in their symptoms as well as a decrease in asthma medication use.

Advances in the management of pediatric asthma, including biologics, offer practitioners the ability to tailor therapies to individual patients. However, asthma treatment guidelines have not kept up with current studies. This review explores the current literature incorporating the use of phenotyping in pediatric patients with asthma to provide precision therapy. Biomarkers can be used to more accurately predict the development of asthma, identify features that may be associated with difficult-to-control or severe asthma, and forecast response to therapies. Biomarkers and other phenotypic data can also be helpful in patients with uncontrolled, severe asthma in the selection of a biologic therapy.

Asthma exacerbations are a significant cause of health care use and mortality. Home management strategies may be effective in managing many exacerbations before presentation to a health care institution. This article focuses on the variety of options available to patients and providers to choose from as they customize an asthma self-management plan. Literature regarding short-acting bronchodilators is reviewed along with studies on more controversial therapies, such as use of home oral steroids, inhaled corticosteroid and beta agonist combination therapy, and macrolides in acute asthma exacerbations.

David R. Stukus

The Internet has forever changed the manner in which we communicate with one another and gather information. Patients and the general public are using online search engines to look for information pertaining to their own health as well as the health of friends and relatives. Unfortunately, the information they encounter is often incorrect and potentially harmful. Many of the sites offering misinformation directly profit by selling nonvalidated tests or treatment options. More than ever, it is important for medical professionals to be aware of the misinformation their patients are encountering online and develop conversations to address this during individual encounters.

IMMUNOLOGY AND ALLERGY CLINICS OF NORTH AMERICA

FORTHCOMING ISSUES

February 2020
Update on Immunotherapy for
Aeroallergens, Foods, and Venoms
Linda S. Cox and Anna Nowak-Wegrzyn,
Editors

May 2020
Rhinosinusitis
Sandra Y. Lin, *Editor*

August 2020
Immunodeficiencies
Mark Ballow and Elena Perez, *Editors*

RECENT ISSUES

August 2019
Infections and Asthma
Mitchell H. Grayson, *Editor*

May 2019
Asthma in Childhood
Leonard B. Bacharier and
Theresa W. Guilbert, *Editors*

February 2019
Primary Immunodeficiency Disorders
Lisa J. Kobrynski, *Editor*

SERIES OF RELATED INTEREST

Pediatric Clinics of North America
Available at: https://www.pediatric.theclinics.com/

THE CLINICS ARE AVAILABLE ONLINE!
Access your subscription at:
www.theclinics.com

Foreword

Pediatric Allergy: The Key to an Evolving Renaissance in Our Specialty

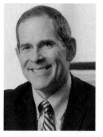

Stephen A. Tilles, MD
Consulting Editor

Historically, pediatric allergic diseases have been understudied, and their treatments were missing their mark. For example, not very many decades ago "parentectomy" was a viable therapeutic option when treating severe pediatric asthma. Subsequently, the concept of asthma as an inflammatory disease emerged, and we began using inhaled corticosteroids (ICS) with the thought that using them regularly would interrupt disease progression and even reverse underlying asthma. To prove this, in the early 1990s, the National Institutes of Health initiated the CAMP ("Child Asthma Management Program") study, boldly randomizing children as young as 5 years old to long-term continuous ICS therapy. We now know that by age 5 "the cat is out of the bag," so to speak, as ICS had no effect on the natural history of asthma.

Meanwhile, we have learned a tremendous amount about the genetics and epigenetics of atopy, asthma, and other allergic diseases, such as food allergy. This has led to more innovative therapeutic and even preventive strategies. For example, the LEAP ("Learning About Peanut Allergy") study demonstrated that introducing regular peanut consumption in the first year of life can prevent high-risk infants from developing peanut allergy. In addition, the recently launched PARK ("Preventing Asthma in High-Risk Kids") study seeks to prevent asthma by treating children as young as age 24 months with omalizumab, a monoclonal antibody directed against immunoglobulin E.

Dr Tilles' consultant work for this issue of *Immunology and Allergy Clinics of North America* was completed before he became an employee of Aimmune Therapeutics.

Immunol Allergy Clin N Am 39 (2019) xi–xii
https://doi.org/10.1016/j.iac.2019.08.002
0889-8561/19/© 2019 Published by Elsevier Inc.

Following both enlightening basic science advances and a long period of disappointing results, biologics such as omalizumab and dupilumab are starting to revolutionize treatment of refractory allergic diseases, such as asthma, urticaria, atopic dermatitis, and food allergy. At the same time, terms such as "personalized medicine" and "precision medicine" have emerged, reflecting the heterogeneity of disease expression, the importance of involving patients and their families in decision making, and the pharmacoeconomic complexity of implementing expensive therapeutic innovations in our health care system.

In this issue of *Immunology and Allergy Clinics of North America*, David Stukus has organized a series of practical reviews authored by experts, who have written thoughtfully and from the patient's perspective. I recommend this issue to all practicing allergists as well as generalists who regularly see children with allergic diseases.

Stephen A. Tilles, MD
Medical Affairs
Aimmune Therapeutics
8000 Marina Boulevard #200
Brisbane, CA 94005, USA

University of Washington
Seattle, WA 98105, USA

E-mail address:
stilles@aimmune.com

Preface
Focusing on Children

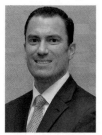

David R. Stukus, MD
Editor

Allergy and Immunology is a unique specialty for many reasons. Unfortunately, many allergic conditions are chronic, with initial presentation during childhood that can last through adulthood. Allergic conditions are also prevalent among the general population. As such, medical providers from across the spectrum must be versed on the recognition and management of these common conditions. This issue of *Immunology and Allergy Clinics of North America* addresses the spectrum of allergic diseases with a focus on the pediatric population.

As the old adage states, "Kids are NOT little adults." Children can present with unique aspects of allergic conditions and require a different approach to diagnosis and management. We have seen recent breakthroughs in the phenotyping of asthma, food allergy, and even allergic rhinitis. Management strategies have changed, and new evidence has helped us appreciate new use of biologic agents to treat asthma, chronic urticaria, and atopic dermatitis. However, one of the most exciting areas pertaining to pediatric allergy is in the realm of prevention. Wouldn't it be magnificent if we could accurately identify those babies at highest risk to develop atopy and offer concrete advice to expecting parents on measures they can take to prevent their child from going down the Th2 path?

Our issue begins with an up-to-date summary of the evidence surrounding prevention strategies. Providers can use this information during discussion with parents and can now actively recommend specific measures to help prevent atopic dermatitis or food allergy development. There are several articles that discuss practical application of current guidelines and how providers can implement best practices for their patients, including early peanut introduction, guidance regarding the management of younger siblings of food-allergic children, utilization of oral food challenges in the office setting, and realistic approaches to children with allergies to only 1 or 2 nuts. Atopic dermatitis can be frustrating for parents due to the recurrent nature of this chronic skin condition, and 2 articles offer thorough information surrounding causes,

Immunol Allergy Clin N Am 39 (2019) xiii–xiv
https://doi.org/10.1016/j.iac.2019.08.001
0889-8561/19/© 2019 Published by Elsevier Inc.

immunology.theclinics.com

contributing factors, and approaches to therapy. Widespread newborn screening for severe combined immune deficiency represents one of the great advances in our specialty, but questions arise when results come back abnormal, a situation addressed in depth in this issue. There are also 3 articles that provide roadmaps for approaching the diagnosis and treatment of children with vocal cord dysfunction and asthma. Last, we live in a brave new world, and our families all come to us already armed with information and preconceived notions about their child's health. It is up to all of us to understand not only where they are getting their information from but also how to have conversations addressing the misinformation they often encounter online.

As you read through this issue, keeping a historical approach in mind can offer a fun and rewarding glimpse into how far we have come in regards to the prevention, diagnosis, and management of various allergic conditions. It's exciting to appreciate that none of these articles could have been written 10 or even 5 years ago. It's even more exciting to think about what discoveries the next 5 or 10 years will bring.

David R. Stukus, MD
Division of Allergy and Immunology
Nationwide Children's Hospital
The Ohio State University College of Medicine
700 Children's Drive
Columbus, OH 43205, USA

E-mail address:
david.stukus@nationwidechildrens.org

It's Not Mom's Fault
Prenatal and Early Life Exposures that Do and Do Not Contribute to Food Allergy Development

Elissa M. Abrams, MD[a], Edmond S. Chan, MD[b],*

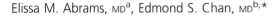

KEYWORDS

• Food allergy • Food allergy prevention • Peanut allergy

KEY POINTS

• The most effective preventative strategy to date has been early allergenic solid introduction, in particular egg, peanut, and (potentially) cow's milk.
• There is insufficient evidence to support use of hydrolyzed formula as a means of allergy prevention.
• Early skin moisturization may be effective for eczema prevention in infancy (which by extension may have a role in food allergy prevention).
• Studies on vitamin D, omega 3, and probiotic supplementation; breastfeeding; early dietary diversity; and maternal peanut ingestion during pregnancy and breastfeeding are inconsistent.

INTRODUCTION

Food allergy is estimated to affect 2% to 10% of the population worldwide, and there has been an increase in food allergy prevalence over time.[1] Some food allergies, such as peanut allergy, are rarely outgrown.[2] In addition, food allergy has a very significant effect on quality of life.[3] As a result, there has been an increasing focus on food allergy prevention.

There are several genetic risk factors associated with the development of food allergy, such as a family history of atopy, genetic polymorphisms, sex, and ethnicity.[4]

Disclosure Statement: Both authors are on the medical advisory group for Food Allergy Canada. Dr E.S. Chan has received research support from DBV Technologies, has been a member of advisory boards for Pfizer, Aralez Pharmaceuticals, Pediapharm, and Leo Pharma, and was an expert panel and coordinating committee member of the National Institute of Allergy and Infectious Diseases (NIAID)-sponsored Guidelines for Peanut Allergy Prevention.
[a] Department of Pediatrics, Section of Allergy and Clinical Immunology, University of Manitoba, FE125-685 William Avenue, Winnipeg, Manitoba R2A 5L9, Canada; [b] Department of Pediatrics, Division of Allergy and Immunology, University of British Columbia, BC Children's Hospital, 4480 Oak Street, Vancouver, British Columbia V6H 3V4, Canada
* Corresponding author.
E-mail address: EChan5@cw.bc.ca

Immunol Allergy Clin N Am 39 (2019) 447–457
https://doi.org/10.1016/j.iac.2019.06.001
0889-8561/19/© 2019 Elsevier Inc. All rights reserved.
immunology.theclinics.com

However, it is also thought there are environmental factors that may contribute to food allergy development, thus opening the door for allergy prevention.

The goal of this article is to review prenatal and postnatal environmental exposures that may have a role in food allergy prevention and review the evidence that supports (or refutes) the use of such strategies.

COMBINED PRENATAL AND POSTNATAL EXPOSURES
Maternal Peanut Ingestion in Pregnancy and Breastfeeding

Evidence regarding peanut ingestion in pregnancy is conflicting and limited to observational studies. A systematic review on the influence of prenatal and early childhood peanut exposure in 2010 noted that the evidence was "heterogeneous" and "limited in quality" which "hindered the development of definitive conclusions."[5]

Several retrospective studies have demonstrated an increased risk of peanut sensitization and/or allergy in childhood with increased maternal peanut ingestion. For example, a case control study of 403 infants with diagnosed peanut allergy compared with age-matched nonatopic controls found that maternal peanut consumption in pregnancy was significantly higher in the peanut allergic group (odds ratio [OR] 4.22, 95% CI 1.57–11.30).[6] In contrast, a few studies have found no association between maternal peanut ingestion and risk of peanut allergy in childhood.[7]

Several recent observational studies have documented a decreased risk of peanut allergy with increased maternal peanut ingestion in pregnancy. For example, in contrast to previous retrospective studies, a large prospective national cohort study (Growing Up Today Study 2) of 10,907 mothers and their children documented a strong inverse association between compared peripregnancy peanut or tree nut consumption ($\geq$5 times vs <1 time per month) and physician-diagnosed peanut or tree nut allergy in childhood (OR 0.31, 95% CI 0.13–0.75).[8]

A recent secondary analysis of a nested cohort within the 1995 Canadian Asthma Primary Prevention Study also suggests that maternal peanut consumption while breastfeeding (in combination with early peanut ingestion in infancy) may reduce the risk of peanut allergy.[9] Of 342 families within this cohort, the lowest incidence of peanut sensitization (1.7%) was observed among children whose mothers consumed peanuts while breastfeeding and introduced peanuts into the diets of their infants by 1 year of age. Incidence of peanut allergy was significantly higher ($P<.05$) if mothers avoided peanuts while breastfeeding, even if peanut was introduced directly into the infant diet by 1 year of age (17.6%).

There are several possible reasons for the discrepancies in the literature, which highlight the limitations of the studies to date. The older retrospective studies largely had an outcome of peanut sensitization, in contrast to the newer prospective studies with oral challenge–proven peanut allergy, and are limited by recall bias. Other factors (eg, atopic status; peanut consumption while breastfeeding; environmental exposure; and duration, frequency, and exposure level of antigen) may play a role.

Avoiding peanut consumption in pregnancy and breastfeeding is not without potential harms. A Cochrane Review on maternal dietary antigen avoidance during pregnancy, although not looking specifically at peanuts, found that antigen-avoidance diets were associated with a significantly lower mean gestational weight gain, nonsignificant higher risk of preterm birth, and a nonsignificant reduction in mean birthweight, while also noting no significant reduction in atopic disease.[10]

Current guidelines do not recommend peanut avoidance in pregnancy or breastfeeding as a means of peanut allergy prevention.[11,12] In the future, there may be a protective role for peanut consumption, although randomized studies are required.

Omega 3 Supplementation

Omega 3 supplementation has an antiinflammatory role through eicosapentaenoic acid, which has been postulated to have an effect on the risk of food allergy. However, studies to date have conflicting results. Some studies on omega 3 supplementation have looked specifically at supplementation in pregnancy, whereas others have looked at the antenatal and postnatal period as well.

For example, the Docosahexaenoic Acid to Optimize Mother Infant Outcome (DOMInO) study randomized 706 pregnant mothers to fish oil capsules from 21 weeks gestation until birth or to placebo (vegetable oil capsules) and found no significant difference in food allergy at 1 year of age between the omega-supplementation and control groups (absolute risk reduction 0.70, 95% CI 0.45–1.09, $P = .12$).[13]

A systematic review and meta-analysis of omega 3 and 6 oils for primary prevention of allergic disease found "no clear evidence of benefit" for reduced risk of allergic sensitization (risk ratio [RR] food allergy 0.51, 95% CI 0.10–2.55).[14] In contrast, a more recent systematic review and meta-analysis on diet during pregnancy and risk of allergic disease found that, based on 6 studies, fish oil supplementation during pregnancy and lactation may reduce risk of egg sensitization (RR 0.69, 95% CI 0.53–0.90).[10]

At this time, based on conflicting evidence to date, there is no firm evidence that omega supplementation reduces the risk of food allergy.

Probiotics

The data on probiotic supplementation in pregnancy and lactation are not consistent and, to date, have not demonstrated a strong reduction in food allergy outcomes. For example, randomized trial of 1223 pregnant women to probiotics or placebo from 36 weeks gestation until birth noted no difference in atopic disease between the groups, although in the subset with caesarean-sections there was some protection against eczema noted.[15]

There have been some data suggesting that probiotic supplementation may have a role in prevention of eczema. For example, a randomized controlled trial of 1223 pregnant women supplemented with probiotics or placebo from 2 to 4 weeks before delivery until age 6 months in infancy found a significant reduction in eczema (OR 0.74, 95% CI 0.55–9.98, $P = .035$), although no effect on other atopic outcomes was observed.[16] A meta-analysis and systematic review also noted that probiotic supplementation during pregnancy and lactation may reduce risk of eczema (RR 0.78, 95% CI 0.68–0.90).[10]

Limitations to the literature to date include varying intervals of probiotic supplementation, different microorganisms in the probiotics, and varying definitions of allergic outcomes (predominantly including a reliance on sensitization). At this time, as noted in a Cochrane review on the topic, there is "'insufficient evidence" to recommend the addition of probiotics to infants to prevent allergic diseases or food allergy.[17]

POSTNATAL EXPOSURES
Early Moisturization

There is emerging evidence that eczema is due to skin barrier dysfunction and that food sensitization can occur through the skin.[18] Mutations in the filaggrin (FLG) gene (involved in skin hydration and water retention) have been strongly linked with eczema and independently with food allergy as well.[19] It is hypothesized that this association may explain the concept of transcutaneous sensitization to foods.[7]

In keeping with this hypothesis, recent randomized controlled trials of infants at high risk of eczema due to parental atopy found that regular emollient therapy for the first several months of life significantly reduced the incidence of eczema compared with no emollient use.[20,21] One of these studies looked at rates of egg sensitization as a secondary outcome and found no significantly reduced rate.[21] In contrast, a third randomized controlled trial of twice daily ceramide emollient application for the first 6 months of life found a trend toward reduced eczema and food sensitization at both 6 and 12 months of age.[22] It has been shown that emollient use decreases skin pH and increases the proportion of *Streptococcus salivarius* long-term, which may be the cause of this protective effect.[23]

At this time, more long-term evidence is needed for the outcome of food allergy, but there is some preliminary evidence for eczema prevention. Moreover, early regular emollient use is a noninvasive, inexpensive intervention and, as a result, may be considered, especially in higher risk infants.

Breastfeeding

The data on breastfeeding as a food allergy prevention strategy are mixed. Some studies demonstrate a reduced risk of food allergy with breastfeeding.[24] Some studies demonstrate no association between breastfeeding duration and food allergy. For example, the Copenhagen Prospective Study on Asthma in Childhood (COPSAC) noted that among 335 children there was no significant association between duration of exclusive breastfeeding and development of sensitization in the first 6 years of life (OR 0.96, 95% CI 0.84–1.10 at 6 years of age).[25]

The limitations to the literature on breastfeeding include entirely observational studies that have nonuniform breastfeeding durations and variable diagnostic criteria for food allergy (including often relying on food sensitization). Exclusive breastfeeding for the first 4 to 6 months of age is recommended for many other reasons, although current guidelines note no consistent benefit as a means of food allergy prevention.[11]

Use of Hydrolyzed Formula

Guidelines have recommended the use of hydrolyzed formula in high-risk infants when mothers could not, or chose not, to breastfeed as a means of food allergy prevention.[11,12] This was partially based on a Cochrane review that noted "limited evidence" that hydrolyzed formula compared with regular cow's milk formula reduced the risk of infant and childhood allergy and cow's milk allergy.[26,27]

However, a recent meta-analysis of 37 studies (>19,000 participants) noted no evidence that partially or extensively hydrolyzed formulas reduced the risk of any allergic outcomes, including food allergy, and noted a high degree of bias in published studies.[28]

In light of this recent meta-analysis, current evidence does not support the use of hydrolyzed formulas as a means of allergy prevention. Guidelines are beginning to reflect this emerging evidence.[29] These formulas are also potentially expensive and not well tolerated.

Early Introduction of Allergenic Solids

Both observational and randomized controlled trials published over the last decade have supported early introduction of allergenic solids, in particular, peanut, egg, and cow's milk, as a means of food allergy prevention.

The first study to suggest a reduction in peanut allergy with early peanut introduction was a questionnaire-based survey in 2008 that found a higher rate of peanut allergy among 5171 Jewish schoolchildren in the United Kingdom compared with 5615

Jewish schoolchildren in Israel (1.85% vs 0.17%, P<.001).[30] This reduced prevalence was attributed to earlier and more frequent peanut ingestion in the first year of life in Israel compared with the United Kingdom. This study was followed by the Learning Early About Peanut (LEAP) study of 640 infants with either severe eczema and/or egg allergy that demonstrated that early peanut introduction between 4 to 11 months of age reduced the risk of peanut allergy by up to 81% compared with avoidance until 5 years of age.[31] The LEAP study noted a preventative effect in both skin-test negative infants (13.7% vs 1.9%, P<.001) and skin-test positive infants (35.3% vs 10.6%, P = .004), supporting early peanut introduction as a means of both primary and secondary prevention.

The data on early egg introduction are more mixed. The HealthNuts observational study noted that among 2589 infants introduction of eggs at 4 to 6 months of age was associated with a lower prevalence of egg allergy compared with later introduction in both high-risk infants (adjusted OR [aOR] 1.6 for introduction at 10–12 months and 3.4 for introduction after 12 months) and lower risk infants (OR 3.3, 95% CI 1.1–1.9 at 10–12 months).[32] In addition, the PETIT study out of Japan randomized 147 infants with eczema to introduction of heated (cooked) egg powder at 6 months of age or avoidance until 1 year and noted a significantly lower rate of egg allergy with earlier introduction (RR 0.222, 95% CI 0.081–0.607, P = .0012).[33] In fact, the study was so successful that it was halted prematurely.

In contrast, several randomized controlled trials examining early pasteurized raw egg introduction have either not shown a significant effect and/or have shown a high rate of adverse events. The Beating Egg Allergy Trial (BEAT) randomized 319 infants at high risk due to family history of atopic disease to pasteurized egg white at 4 months of age or placebo until 8 months of age and found a significant reduction in egg white sensitization at 1 year of age with early egg introduction (OR 0.46, 95% CI 0.22–0.95), although there was a nonsignificant trend in reduction of egg allergy and a high rate of reactions with early introduction.[34–37] The Solids Timing for Allergy Research (STAR) trial randomized 86 infants with moderate-to-severe eczema to pasteurized raw egg introduction at either 4 months or avoidance until 8 months, with an outcome of egg allergy at 1 year of age. There was a nonsignificant trend toward lower rates of egg allergy in the early introduction group (33%) compared with the control group (51%); relative risk 0.65, 95% CI 0.38–1.11, P = .11), although a high rate of allergic reactions (31%) were noted upon early introduction. It has been postulated that the marked differences in study results may be attributed to the form of egg introduced because studies on early cooked egg introduction have found early ingestion to be protective, whereas studies on early raw egg introduction have either found no significant protective effect and/or a high rate of reactions.

A recent meta-analysis and systematic review of timing of allergenic food introduction and risk of allergic disease found that there was moderate-certainty evidence (5 trials, 1915 participants) that early egg introduction at 4 to 6 months of age was associated with reduced egg allergy (RR 0.56, 95% CI 0.36–0.87) and moderate-certainty evidence (2 trials, 1550 participants) that early peanut introduction at 4 to 11 months of age was associated with reduced peanut allergy (RR 0.29, 95% CI 0.11–0.74).[38]

The studies on early cow's milk introduction have all been observational and supported the potential protective role of early cow's milk introduction. A prospective study of 13,019 infants noted that regular exposure to cow's milk formula starting within the first 14 days of life was associated with a lower risk of immunoglobulin (Ig)-E–mediated cow's milk allergy compared with later exposure (OR 19.3 for introduction after 14 days of age).[39,40] A recent analysis of the HealthNuts longitudinal, population-based study of 5276 infants noted that early exposure to cow's milk within the first 3 months of life was associated with a reduced risk of cow's milk allergy (aOR 0.31, 95% CI 0.10–0.91) at 1 year of age.[41]

There have not been many studies examining the effect of early introduction of other commonly allergenic foods such as wheat, finned fish, shellfish, tree nuts, sesame, or soy. The Enquiring About Tolerance (EAT) study is the only randomized controlled trial to examine early (3 vs 6 months) introduction of multiple allergenic solids (peanut, cow's milk, sesame, whitefish, wheat, cooked egg) in general population infants.[42] In the intention-to-treat analysis, there was no significant difference in the rate of food allergy between the early and standard introduction groups (5.6% vs 7.1%, respectively, P = .32), although in the per-protocol analysis there was a significant reduction in food allergy overall with early introduction (2.4% vs 7.3%, P=.01). In the per-protocol analysis there was a 75% reduction in egg allergy (1.4% vs 5.5%, P=.009) and 100% reduction in peanut allergy (0% vs 2.5%, P=.003) with early intro- duction. Compliance was a significant issue in this study (42.8% overall).

There remain many ongoing questions about early feeding, including the duration that ingestion is required to ensure ongoing tolerance. The only study thus far to examine this is the LEAP-ON study, which examined whether avoidance of peanuts for 1 year after completion of the LEAP study would increase peanut allergy rates. It demonstrated that among 550 of the original LEAP study participants, 1 year of peanut avoidance resulted in no significant increase in the prevalence of peanut allergy among participants in the early introduction group (P = .25).[43,44] The optimal dose of allergen that should be ingested remains unknown, although results from the EAT study have suggested that mean weekly consumption of 2 g a week of peanuts and eggs is effective at reducing the probability of egg or peanut allergy.[42] It remains un- known how frequently these allergens should be ingested, and very few studies have been done in general population infants. A theoretic risk has also been raised that early introduction of allergenic foods may increase the risk of non–IgE-mediated food allergy such as food protein–induced enterocolitis syndrome (FPIES).

Since the release of the LEAP study results, the National Institute of Allergy and In- fectious Diseases expert panel released addendum guidelines for the prevention of peanut allergy in the United States.[45] These addendum guidelines recommend that in high-risk infants (ie, those with severe eczema and/or egg allergy), peanuts should be introduced as early as age 4 to 6 months. Other international guidelines support the introduction of other allergenic foods such as cooked egg at around 6 months but not before 4 months of age.[29,46]

In conclusion, in high-risk infants there is level 1 evidence for earlier introduction of allergenic foods, in particular to cooked eggs and peanuts. There are observa- tional studies that support early cow's milk introduction. Ongoing exposure is as important as age of introduction. Extrapolation from the EAT and HealthNuts studies suggest that early exposure would be effective in general population infants as well. However, significant barriers exist, in particular when considering preemptive testing before introduction (eg, overinterpretation of positive skin prick tests or spe- cific IgE blood tests, and poor availability of infant oral food challenges).[47–49] There remain knowledge gaps about early introduction of some allergenic foods such as tree nuts.

Dietary Diversity

Several observational studies have suggested that increased dietary diversity may reduce the risk of food allergy. For example, in 2011, a longitudinal birth cohort of 594 infant–mother pairs in the United States noted that complementary food introduction before age 4 months reduced the risk of peanut sensitization (aOR 0.2, P = .007) and perhaps egg sensitization (if egg-specific IgE $\geq$0.70 kU/L was used as a cutoff; aOR 0.5, P = .022) at age 2 years in children with parents with allergies or asthma.[50]

There are criticisms that the data on dietary diversity lack biologic plausibility. In addition, the studies vary in their definition of food diversity and outcomes are largely sensitization instead of clinical allergy. No randomized controlled trials have been done.

Although the data are few and observational, and hence no firm conclusions can be made, this is another strategy that could be considered due to general lack of harm. However, care must be taken to ensure that inclusion of a long list of diverse nonallergenic foods does not delay the introduction of allergenic foods, which are higher priority for food allergy prevention.

Vitamin D

Studies have linked less geographic or sun exposure to vitamin D to the development of food allergy. Studies have noted that with increasing distance from the equator there is increased risk of food allergy-related hospitalizations and epinephrine autoinjector prescriptions.[51] Vitamin D has been shown to have innate and adaptive immune functions, including suppression of type 2 T helper cell responses. Recent evidence suggests that polymorphisms that lower vitamin D–binding protein (which increases the biologic availability of vitamin D) attenuate the association between low vitamin D levels and food allergy, and provide some biologic plausibility for the role of vitamin D in the development of food allergy.[52]

In 2013, data from the Australian HealthNuts study of 5276 infants noted that infants of Australian-born parents who had vitamin D insufficiency were significantly more likely to have challenge-proven peanut and/or egg allergy (aOR 11.51, 95% CI 2.01–65.79 and aOR 3.79, 95% CI 1.19–12.08, respectively) and to have multiple (vs single) food allergy, than those without vitamin D insufficiency.[53] However, a more recent case-cohort study of 1074 infants noted no association between vitamin D

Table 1
Exposures and their contribution to food allergy prevention

Exposure	Does Contribute	Does Not Contribute	Highest Level of Evidence	Quality of Evidence
Maternal peanut ingestion during pregnancy and breastfeeding	—	+	Observational	B
Omega 3 supplementation	—	++	RCT	C
Probiotics	—	+	RCT	C
Early moisturization	++		RCT	C
Breastfeeding	—	++	Observational	B
Hydrolyzed formula	—	+++	Observational	B
Early allergenic solid introduction	+++	—	RCT	A
Dietary diversity	—	+	Observational	B
Vitamin D supplementation	—	+	Observational	B

Quality of evidence: A, further research unlikely to change this recommendation; B, further research is likely to have an impact on the authors' confidence in this recommendation; C, further research is very likely to have an important impact on the authors' confidence in this estimate of effect.[56]

Abbreviation: RCT, randomized controlled trial.

insufficiency at birth or 6 months of age and food allergy prevalence (predominantly egg allergy) at 1 year of age.[54]

There are limitations to the literature to date, including variations in the definition of vitamin D insufficiency, known racial differences in vitamin D absorption, the role that atopy (or atopic risk) may play, and differences in vitamin D bioavailability from supplementation versus sun exposure. To date, no randomized studies have been completed and further data are needed. Studies are ongoing, including the VITALITY study, which is the first double-blind randomized controlled trial to examine whether vitamin D supplementation in breastfed infants could decrease the risk of challenge-proven food allergy.[55] Until such time, no formal recommendation about vitamin D supplementation can be made.

SUMMARY

To date, the most effective preventative strategy has been early allergenic solid introduction, in particular egg, peanut, and (potentially) cow's milk (**Table 1**). Early skin moisturization in infancy may be effective for eczema prevention (which theoretically could then prevent food allergy) and seems to be relatively easy to implement. The data on maternal peanut ingestion in pregnancy and breastfeeding are conflicting. Studies on vitamin D, omega 3 and probiotic supplementation, breastfeeding, and early dietary diversity are inconsistent. There is lack of evidence to support the use of hydrolyzed formulas as a means of allergy prevention. It is not known at this time whether breastfeeding has any role in food allergy prevention. Ongoing studies to further delineate possible environmental modifications in pregnancy, or early infancy, may help alleviate the ongoing burden of food allergy in children.

REFERENCES

1. Chafen JJS, Newberry SJ, Riedl MA, et al. Diagnosing and managing common food allergies: a systematic review. JAMA 2010;303:1848–56.
2. Sicherer SH, Sampson HA. Food allergy. J Allergy Clin Immunol 2010;125: S116–25.
3. Gupta RS, Springston EE, Smith B, et al. Food allergy knowledge, attitudes, and beliefs of parents with food-allergic children in the United States. Pediatr Allergy Immunol 2010;21:927–34.
4. Asai Y, Eslami A, van Ginkel CD, et al. Genome-wide association study and meta-analysis in multiple populations identifies new loci for peanut allergy and establishes C11orf30/EMSY as a genetic risk factor for food allergy. J Allergy Clin Immunol 2018;141(3):991–1001.
5. Thompson RL, Miles LM, Lunn J, et al. Peanut sensitisation and allergy: influence of early life exposure to peanuts. Br J Nutr 2010;103:1278–86.
6. DesRoches A, Infante-Rivard C, Paradis L, et al. Peanut allergy: is maternal transmission of antigens during pregnancy and breastfeeding a risk factor? J Investig Allergol Clin Immunol 2010;20:289–94.
7. Lack G, Fox D, Northstone K, et al. Factors associated with the development of peanut allergy in childhood. N Engl J Med 2003;348:977–85.
8. Frazier AL, Camargo CAJ, Malspeis S, et al. Prospective study of peripregnancy consumption of peanuts or tree nuts by mothers and the risk of peanut or tree nut allergy in their offspring. JAMA Pediatr 2014;168:156–62.
9. Pitt TJ, Becker AB, Chan-Yeung M, et al. Reduced risk of peanut sensitization following exposure through breast-feeding and early peanut introduction. J Allergy Clin Immunol 2018;141:620–5.e1.

10. Garcia-Larsen V, Ierodiakonou D, Jarrold K, et al. Diet during pregnancy and infancy and risk of allergic or autoimmune disease: a systematic review and meta-analysis. PLoS Med 2018;15:e1002507.

11. Fleischer DM, Spergel JM, Assa'ad AH, et al. Primary prevention of allergic disease through nutritional interventions. J Allergy Clin Immunol Pract 2013;1:29–36.

12. Chan ES, Cummings C. Dietary exposures and allergy prevention in high-risk infants: a joint statement with the Canadian Society of Allergy and Clinical Immunology. Paediatr Child Health 2013;18:545–54.

13. Palmer DJ, Sullivan T, Gold MS, et al. Effect of n-3 long chain polyunsaturated fatty acid supplementation in pregnancy on infants' allergies in first year of life: randomised controlled trial. BMJ 2012;344:e184.

14. Anandan C, Nurmatov U, Sheikh A. Omega 3 and 6 oils for primary prevention of allergic disease: systematic review and meta-analysis. Allergy 2009;64:840–8.

15. Kallio S, Kukkonen AK, Savilahti E, et al. Perinatal probiotic intervention prevented allergic disease in a Caesarean-delivered subgroup at 13-year follow-up. Clin Exp Allergy 2019;49(4):506–15.

16. Kukkonen K, Savilahti E, Haahtela T, et al. Probiotics and prebiotic galacto-oligosaccharides in the prevention of allergic diseases: a randomized, double-blind, placebo-controlled trial. J Allergy Clin Immunol 2007;119:192–8.

17. Osborn DA, Sinn JK. Probiotics in infants for prevention of allergic disease and food hypersensitivity. Cochrane Database Syst Rev 2007;(4):CD006475.

18. Schneider L, Tilles S, Lio P, et al. Atopic dermatitis: a practice parameter update 2012. J Allergy Clin Immunol 2013;131:227–95.

19. Irvine AD, McLean WHI, Leung DYM. Filaggrin mutations associated with skin and allergic diseases. N Engl J Med 2011;365:1315–27.

20. Simpson EL, Chalmers JR, Hanifin JM, et al. Emollient enhancement of the skin barrier from birth offers effective atopic dermatitis prevention. J Allergy Clin Immunol 2014;134:818–23.

21. Horimukai K, Morita K, Narita M, et al. Application of moisturizer to neonates prevents development of atopic dermatitis. J Allergy Clin Immunol 2014;134:824–30.e6.

22. Lowe AJ, Su JC, Allen KJ, et al. A randomized trial of a barrier lipid replacement strategy for the prevention of atopic dermatitis and allergic sensitization: the PEBBLES pilot study. Br J Dermatol 2018;178:e19–21.

23. Glatz M, Jo J-H, Kennedy EA, et al. Emollient use alters skin barrier and microbes in infants at risk for developing atopic dermatitis. PLoS One 2018;13:e0192443.

24. van Odijk J, Kull I, Borres MP, et al. Breastfeeding and allergic disease: a multidisciplinary review of the literature (1966-2001) on the mode of early feeding in infancy and its impact on later atopic manifestations. Allergy 2003;58:833–43.

25. Jelding-Dannemand E, Malby Schoos A-M, Bisgaard H. Breast-feeding does not protect against allergic sensitization in early childhood and allergy-associated disease at age 7 years. J Allergy Clin Immunol 2015;136:1302–13.

26. Osborn DA, Sinn J. Formulas containing hydrolysed protein for prevention of allergy and food intolerance in infants. Cochrane Database Syst Rev 2006;(4):CD003664.

27. Zutavern A, Brockow I, Schaaf B, et al. Timing of solid food introduction in relation to eczema, asthma, allergic rhinitis, and food and inhalant sensitization at the age of 6 years: results from the prospective birth cohort study LISA. Pediatrics 2008;121:e44–52.

28. Boyle RJ, Ierodiakonou D, Khan T, et al. Hydrolysed formula and risk of allergic or autoimmune disease: systematic review and meta-analysis. BMJ 2016;352:i974.

29. Netting MJ, Campbell DE, Koplin JJ. An Australian Consensus on infant feeding guidelines to prevent food allergy: outcomes from the Australian infant feeding Summit. J Allergy Clin Immunol Pract 2017;5:1617–24.

30. Du Toit G, Katz Y, Sasieni P, et al. Early consumption of peanuts in infancy is associated with a low prevalence of peanut allergy. J Allergy Clin Immunol 2008;122: 984–91.

31. Du Toit G, Roberts G, Sayre PH, et al. Randomized trial of peanut consumption in infants at risk for peanut allergy. N Engl J Med 2015;372:803–13.

32. Koplin JJ, Osborne NJ, Wake M, et al. Can early introduction of egg prevent egg allergy in infants? A population-based study. J Allergy Clin Immunol 2010;126: 807–13.

33. Natsume O, Kabashima S, Nakazato J, et al. Two-step egg introduction for prevention of egg allergy in high-risk infants with eczema (PETIT): a randomised, double-blind, placebo-controlled trial. Lancet 2017;389:276–86.

34. Wei-Liang Tan J, Valerio C, Barnes EH, et al. A randomized trial of egg introduction from 4 months of age in infants at risk for egg allergy. J Allergy Clin Immunol 2017;139:1621–8.e8.

35. Palmer DJ, Metcalfe J, Makrides M, et al. Early regular egg exposure in infants with eczema: a randomized controlled trial. J Allergy Clin Immunol 2013;132: 387–92.e1.

36. Palmer DJ, Sullivan TR, Gold MS, et al. Randomized controlled trial of early regular egg intake to prevent egg allergy. J Allergy Clin Immunol 2017;139: 1600–7.e2.

37. Bellach J, Schwarz V, Ahrens B, et al. Randomized placebo-controlled trial of hen's egg consumption for primary prevention in infants. J Allergy Clin Immunol 2017;139:1591–9.e2.

38. Ierodiakonou D, Garcia-Larsen V, Logan A, et al. Timing of allergenic food introduction to the infant diet and risk of allergic or autoimmune disease: a systematic review and meta-analysis. JAMA 2016;316:1181–92.

39. Katz Y, Rajuan N, Goldberg MR, et al. Early exposure to cow's milk protein is protective against IgE-mediated cow's milk protein allergy. J Allergy Clin Immunol 2010;126:77–82.e1.

40. Onizawa Y, Noguchi E, Okada M, et al. The association of the delayed introduction of cow's milk with ige-mediated cow's milk allergies. J Allergy Clin Immunol Pract 2016;4:481–8.e2.

41. Peters RL, Koplin JJ, Dharmage SC, et al. Early exposure to cow's milk protein is associated with a reduced risk of cow's milk allergic outcomes. J Allergy Clin Immunol Pract 2019;7(2):462–70.e1.

42. Perkin MR, Logan K, Tseng A, et al. Randomized trial of introduction of allergenic foods in breast-fed infants. N Engl J Med 2016;374:1733–43.

43. Du Toit G, Sayre PH, Roberts G, et al. Effect of avoidance on peanut allergy after early peanut consumption. N Engl J Med 2016;374:1435–43.

44. Nowak-Wegrzyn A, Chehade M, Groetch ME, et al. International consensus guidelines for the diagnosis and management of food protein-induced enterocolitis syndrome: executive summary-Workgroup Report of the Adverse Reactions to Foods Committee, American Academy of Allergy, Asthma & Immunology. J Allergy Clin Immunol 2017;139:1111–26.e4.

45. Togias A, Cooper SF, Acebal ML, et al. Addendum guidelines for the prevention of peanut allergy in the United States: report of the National Institute of Allergy and Infectious Diseases-sponsored expert panel. J Allergy Clin Immunol 2017; 139:29–44.

46. Preventing food allergy in higher risk infants: guidance for healthcare professionals. Available at: https://www.bsaci.org/pdf/Early-feeding-guidance-for-HCPs.pdf. Accessed April 5, 2019.
47. Turner PJ, Campbell DE. Implementing primary prevention for peanut allergy at a population level. JAMA 2017;317:1111–2.
48. Wood RA, Burks AW. LEAPing forward with the new guidelines. J Allergy Clin Immunol 2017;139:52–3.
49. Abrams EM, Singer AG, Soller L, et al. Knowledge gaps and barriers to early peanut introduction among allergists, pediatricians, and family physicians. J Allergy Clin Immunol Pract 2019;7(2):681–4.
50. Joseph CLM, Ownby DR, Havstad SL, et al. Early complementary feeding and risk of food sensitization in a birth cohort. J Allergy Clin Immunol 2011;127: 1203–10.e5.
51. Mullins RJ, Clark S, Camargo CAJ. Regional variation in epinephrine autoinjector prescriptions in Australia: more evidence for the vitamin D-anaphylaxis hypothesis. Ann Allergy Asthma Immunol 2009;103:488–95.
52. Koplin JJ, Suaini NHA, Vuillermin P, et al. Polymorphisms affecting vitamin D-binding protein modify the relationship between serum vitamin D (25[OH]D3) and food allergy. J Allergy Clin Immunol 2016;137:500–6.e4.
53. Allen KJ, Koplin JJ, Ponsonby A-L, et al. Vitamin D insufficiency is associated with challenge-proven food allergy in infants. J Allergy Clin Immunol 2013;131: 1109–16, 1116.e1-6.
54. Molloy J, Koplin JJ, Allen KJ, et al. Vitamin D insufficiency in the first 6 months of infancy and challenge-proven IgE-mediated food allergy at 1 year of age: a case-cohort study. Allergy 2017;72:1222–31.
55. Allen KJ, Panjari M, Koplin JJ, et al. VITALITY trial: protocol for a randomised controlled trial to establish the role of postnatal vitamin D supplementation in infant immune health. BMJ Open 2015;5:e009377.
56. GRADE (Grading of recommendations Assessment, development and Evaluation) Working group 2007 1 (modified by the EBM guidelines Editorial Team). Available at: http://www.gradeworkinggroup.org/. Accessed April 5, 2019.

Implementation of Early Peanut Introduction Guidelines: It Takes a Village

Irene J. Mikhail, MD

KEYWORDS

- Peanut allergy • Allergy prevention • Food allergy • Food introduction

KEY POINTS

- Early peanut introduction around 6 months of age is thought to help prevent the development of peanut allergy in high-risk infants.
- It is unclear if high-risk infants need to have peanut allergy testing before first ingestion of peanut.
- Implementing new guidelines related to peanut introduction on a national level has been challenging for several reasons.

INTRODUCTION

Food allergy can affect up to 5% of the pediatric population in the United States.[1] There is special interest in peanut allergy because it is rarely outgrown, is most often associated with fatal anaphylaxis,[2] and has a significant effect on quality of life.[2,3] Currently, there are no Food and Drug Administration–approved treatment options for peanut allergy, although at least 2 potential treatment options are undergoing clinical trials.[4] Although these treatment options appear promising, they are not without risk, complication, and cost. Furthermore, they provide no guarantee of complete tolerance to peanut.[4] Consequently, there has been, and continues to be, great interest in the prevention of peanut allergy.

HISTORICAL PERSPECTIVE

In the late 1990s, partially in response to the growing incidence of food allergy, international organizations released recommendations calling for the avoidance of highly allergenic foods until later in life.[5,6] These recommendations were based on an assumption of the protective role of exclusive breastfeeding, an understanding of mucosal immunity in allergy development and observations on increased rates of eczema when solid food was introduced before 4 months of age.[7] However, an

Disclosure Statement: No disclosures.
Division of Allergy and Immunology, Nationwide Children's Hospital, 700 Children's Drive, Columbus, OH 43205, USA
E-mail address: Irene.mikhail@nationwidechildrens.org

Immunol Allergy Clin N Am 39 (2019) 459–467
https://doi.org/10.1016/j.iac.2019.07.002
0889-8561/19/© 2019 Elsevier Inc. All rights reserved.

understanding of the impact of different routes of sensitization (and preference for oral sensitization to precede other routes of sensitization) began to emerge, and new data began to challenge these recommendations. For instance, a compelling study by Du Toit and colleagues[8] found a pattern in which food allergies were prevalent at a higher rate in London (where peanut avoidance was practiced), compared with Tel Aviv (where peanut consumption began in infancy) in a genetically similar population. In 2008, the American Academy of Pediatrics reversed its original recommendation, indicating the timing of allergic foods should be left up to personal and cultural preferences because there was a lack of evidence to make recommendations in any specific direction.[9] The American Academy of Allergy and Immunology (AAAAI) and Canadian society made similar reversals in 2013.[10,11]

The paucity of evidence on the optimal timing of introduction of peanut lead to the Learning Early About Peanut trial (LEAP), a randomized control trial that compared the incidence of peanut allergy in a group of infants who had deliberate early introduction of peanut with a group of infants who delayed introduction of peanut.[12]

LEARNING EARLY ABOUT PEANUT TRIAL

The results of the LEAP trial were published in February 2015. High-risk infants were defined as those with either an egg allergy or moderate to severe atopic dermatitis. All infants had peanut skin prick testing (SPT) at study entry. Infants with an SPT greater than 4 mm were assumed to be allergic to peanut and were excluded from the trial. The remaining infants were separated into a group with no peanut sensitization and those with SPT of 1 to 4 mm. Each group was then randomized into early introduction, which considered of eating 2 g of peanut product in the form of Bamba, 3 times a week or strict peanut avoidance. Infants in the early introduction group had an oral food challenge (OFC) to peanut before beginning peanut introduction at home. At the end of 5 years, all infants who were randomized had an OFC to peanut.[12]

The results of the LEAP trial were compelling, with an overall risk reduction of peanut allergy from 17.2% in the avoidance group to 3.2% in the introduction group. In the group with no peanut sensitization, there was a relative risk reduction of 86% in children who consumed peanut, compared with those who avoided peanut, showing promising primary prevention. In the sensitized group, there was a 70% relative risk reduction in the consuming group compared with the avoiding group, demonstrating secondary prevention.[12] The LEAP-On trial went on to show that infants who consumed peanut in infancy were able to maintain peanut tolerance, even after they stopped regular peanut consumption, demonstrating they had achieved true peanut tolerance.[13]

Although the LEAP trial demonstrated quite robust data, it left many unanswered questions. How frequent was peanut consumption required to obtain the protective effect? Which population would benefit the most from early introduction? Could the infants who were excluded from the study because of large skin test benefit from early introduction? Do infants need to have allergy testing before eating peanut product? Could the results seen in the study be extrapolated to other populations? Essentially, the message behind the LEAP trial was understood, but there was confusion on how to implement the findings in clinical practice.

NATIONAL INSTITUTES OF HEALTH GUIDELINES: PUBLICATION OF THE ADDENDUM GUIDELINES FROM THE NATIONAL INSTITUTE OF ALLERGY AND INFECTIOUS DISEASES

In response to the compelling data published in the LEAP trial, international experts from pediatrics, allergy/immunology, and dermatology quickly released consensus guidelines to assist with the implementation of the LEAP data.[14] Subsequently, the National Institute of Allergy and Infectious Diseases (NIAID) released more detailed guidelines that made specific recommendations on peanut introduction and testing based on infant risk factors. These guidelines were published in January 2017 and suggested discussing the introduction of peanut between 4 and 6 months of age after other solid foods are introduced for infants with eczema or egg allergy.[15] The guidelines further recommend that high-risk infants, defined as infants with egg allergy or severe atopic dermatitis, should have allergy testing before peanut introduction. The guidelines did not make specific recommendations for infants who do not have eczema or egg allergy, stating they should introduce peanut according to family and cultural preferences.

Although serum-specific immunoglobulin E (IgE) was not found to be very specific in the LEAP trial or in other trials, the guidelines do include the use of serum-specific IgE as a screening tool in some populations, especially when access to an allergist may be limited. Infants with a negative peanut IgE (<0.10 KU/L) have minimal risk for a systemic reaction to peanut and can introduce peanut at home without evaluation by an allergist. However, any value greater than 0.10 KU/L is not very sensitive and would require referral to an allergist for evaluation.[15]

An allergist should evaluate all the high-risk infants (egg allergy or severe atopic dermatitis) who have a serum-specific IgE greater than 0.10 KU/L (when performed) with SPT and OFC. An infant with a peanut SPT less than or equal to 2 has a minimal chance of a systemic reaction and can be instructed to introduce peanut at home. Those with an SPT of 3 to 7 mm warrant further evaluation with an OFC to determine if the infant can tolerate peanut. Infants with an SPT greater than 7 mm have a high likelihood of peanut allergy and should be counseled appropriately. An upper limit of 7 mm was chosen, rather than the 4 mm used in the LEAP trial, based on data from the HealthNuts study, which was a longitudinal, population-based study looking at the incidence of peanut allergy in infants in Australia that included an OFC for all infants.[16]

All infants who are considered tolerant to peanut (either by SPT or passed OFC) should be instructed to maintain peanut in their diet 3 times a week in order to ensure continued tolerance to peanut. As part of the NIAID addendum guidelines, specific recommendations were made on how to introduce peanut protein into an infant's diet. Special interest, of course, was given to the prevention of choking. It is imperative that infants are not given peanuts. Instead, they can be offered peanut butter or peanut-flavored snacks. Peanut butter can be mixed with hot water or mixed in a puree to a consistency the infant is used to eating. Two grams of peanut protein is equal to approximately 2 teaspoons of peanut butter or 21 peanut-flavored snacks. Detailed recipes can be found on the NIAID Web site.[15]

SIBLINGS WITH PEANUT ALLERGY

The guidelines make no recommendations regarding testing infants who have older siblings with peanut allergy. Previous studies have shown that a family history of a sibling with a peanut allergy may slightly increase the risk of peanut allergy.[17–19] However, these studies have several inherent flaws, primarily reliance on self-report or evidence of sensitization to define allergy. Others have noted that siblings of children of peanut allergy are more likely to avoid peanut or to be mislabeled as peanut allergic, potential risk factors for peanut allergy.[20] Gupta and colleagues[21] suggested that siblings of peanut-allergic children did not have a higher incidence of peanut allergy, when allergy was defined as clinical reactivity and sensitization, but were more likely to have evidence of peanut sensitization. Although it is unclear if the potential increased risk of peanut allergy in siblings of children with peanut allergy is genetic[22] or related to environmental responses,[21] their risk of clinically insignificant sensitization is high. Furthermore, other risk factors, such as egg allergy or eczema, seem to be more significant risk factors for the development of peanut allergy. Many believe the slightly higher risk of peanut allergy in siblings of peanut-allergic children is mitigated by earlier peanut introduction. Therefore, screening for peanut allergy is not necessary when an infant has a sibling with peanut allergy and can actually lead to unnecessary delay and food avoidance.

Requiring allergy testing for all infants who have a sibling with peanut allergy, the vast majority of whom would be able to safely tolerate peanut, does not make sense from a public health perspective. However, when allergy testing is available, it can be offered to caregivers who are uncomfortable introducing peanut without testing. Many families are comfortable introducing without testing, especially when the risks are explained. However, in this author's experience, some families refuse to introduce peanut without testing, especially if they have witnessed another child have anaphylaxis to peanut. In these situations, providing allergy tests for reassurance, and OFC when testing is positive, is sometimes necessary to introduce peanut into an infant's diet. However, it is important to note that testing is not required in this situation and counseling against the need for testing is always an option.

Some families have chosen to become strictly peanut-free after 1 member develops a peanut allergy and struggle with the recommendation to keep peanut a regular part of another infant's diet. In these cases, the author recommends that peanut either be introduced into the diet away from home if the child frequents another caregiver's home regularly or be introduced into the home in a safe location for the purpose of remaining in the tolerant child's diet. Especially for infants with a risk factor for developing a peanut allergy, it is important to highlight the recommendation to maintain peanut in the infant's diet.

BREASTFEEDING

Many countries have changed policies to include proactive peanut introduction between 4 and 6 months of age based on the LEAP data. However, others have questioned the wisdom of these global changes, especially when considering developing countries, which may have different risk factors, such as malnutrition and human immunodeficiency virus. To date, all studies have been conducted in developed countries. Levin and colleagues[23] advise the risks associated with weaning be balanced against the risk of developing a peanut allergy and encourage recommendations be country specific. It is important to note, however, that in the studies that have been done investigating early introduction of allergenic foods, the introduction of peanut did not hinder breastfeeding rates or duration.[12,13,24]

BARRIERS TO IMPLEMENTATION

Although the NIAID guidelines were published in 2017, bringing the guidelines into widespread clinical practice has been met with several barriers. In a survey conducted 3 months after the guidelines were released (and 26 months after the LEAP data were published), Greenhawt and colleagues[25] found that caregivers and expectant caregivers were very hesitant to adopt these recommended changes, with only 30% of nationally surveyed participants indicating a willingness to introduce peanut to an infant around 6 months of age. The survey conducted was a nationally represented (other than age, gender, and marital status) sample of 1000 expectant caregivers and

1000 new caregivers (mean age, 30.1%; 99.6% women and 79% married). Approximately half of the sample agreed that the timing of food introduction could influence the development of food allergy. However, nearly 40% preferred to wait until after 11 months of age to introduce peanut, and more than half preferred allergy testing and OFC after 11 months of age. Interestingly, respondents with a family history of peanut allergy, including other children with food allergy, did not have any increased willingness to introduce peanut early.[25]

The hesitation to adopt new guidelines likely goes beyond family preferences and extends to physician knowledge and comfort. Abrams and colleagues[26] surveyed allergists, pediatricians, and family practitioners on approach to an infant at risk of developing peanut allergy and found that pediatricians and family practitioners were unclear on the risk factors for infants at high risk of developing peanut allergy, citing a sibling with a peanut allergy as the most important risk factor. In this study, only 24.6%, 3.95%, and 4.22% of allergists, pediatricians, and family practitioners, respectively, recommended preemptive testing for infants with severe eczema before peanut introduction. In an abstract presented at the AAAAI in 2018, the author's group described difficulty in getting pediatric colleagues to refer to a designated early introduction of peanut clinic, designed to address the need to test and challenge high-risk infants in a timely manner, and how the use of a quality improvement algorithm helped to address the difficulty.[27]

Even when guidelines are followed and high-risk infants are appropriately referred for allergy evaluation, performing OFC when needed can be difficult. Stukus and colleagues[28] described the implementation of these guidelines in clinical practice and found that 40% of infants who were told to return for an OFC were lost to follow-up. When infants were challenged on the same day as SPT, a resolution was more likely to be established.

UNANSWERED QUESTIONS
Testing Requirements

Many controversies remain regarding early peanut introduction. Perhaps the most pressing issue is the question of which patients, if any, require testing before introduction. The NIAID addendum guidelines call for testing of high-risk infants, as previously described. Other countries, such as the United Kingdom and Australia, did not include the need for allergy testing in their revised national guidelines.[29,30] Australia's guidelines do not make any recommendations for testing, instead suggesting that all infants be fed peanut in a graded manner around 6 months of age.[29] The United Kingdom has a similar policy as Australia, but does note that allergy referral can be considered for high-risk infants (but should be considered against the potential for delayed introduction).[30]

Concerns about testing relate to the capacity of allergists' to meet the demand. In the HealthNuts study, an estimate of 11% of infants would have met the inclusion criteria of moderate to severe eczema or egg allergy by 6 months of age. With an expected 300,000 births each year, this would equate to 33,000 referrals to allergy for allergy testing. Based on the LEAP trial, approximately 4488 infants would require OFCs. Koplin and colleagues[31] used these data to estimate the feasibility of implementing the LEAP data and concluded there would not be enough allergists in Australia to perform the necessary OFC to adequately implement the NIAID guidelines.

The idea to forgo testing comes from the observation that reactions in the infant population are usually mild. When examining the reactions at baseline OFC in the LEAP data, all the reactions were mild and able to be treated with antihistamine alone. Furthermore, Koplin and colleagues[31] described reactions to first peanut introduction in the HealthNuts study and found there were no anaphylactic reactions in the group that introduced at home. Most of the 150 reactions occurring in the 400 OFC conducted in the office were mild and required either no treatment or treatment with antihistamines. However, there were 6 cases of anaphylaxis that occurred in both high-risk and low-risk infants.[31]

Because systemic reactions requiring epinephrine are rare in the infant population, some believe the requirement for allergy testing before introduction may be leading to an unnecessary delay in peanut introduction and overburdening limited allergy resources. However, others argue that although systemic reactions are rare, they do still occur. On a population level, if all infants are told to introduce peanuts without testing, it is inevitable that some infants will have systemic reactions that families may be unprepared to handle. Not only can this be dangerous for the infant but also it may inadvertently lead to a hesitation to introduce peanut. In a simulated model, Shaker and colleagues[32] found that a no-screening approach was more cost-effective than a screening approach in implementing early peanut introduction, but also led to a greater number of peanut-allergic reactions.

At this time it is unknown if there is a need to screen every high-risk infant and the best screening method. Furthermore, it is unclear if the current screening recommendation is creating a delay in peanut introduction or overburdening the capacity of allergists. However, there have not been any reports indicating an inability to adequately test and challenge high-risk infants. On the contrary, it is far more likely that high-risk infants are being underreferred for allergy evaluation and consequently may not be discussing peanut introduction.[33] It is possible, as the guidelines become more engrained in the culture, that a greater number of high-risk infants will be identified and referred. Given the current reluctance to adopt the new guidelines, there is a concern that primary care providers would be reluctant to encourage early peanut introduction in high-risk infants without prior testing. Further recommendations should take into account primary care physician willingness to comply with the recommendation.

It is desirable to identify the infants who would attain the highest yield from evaluation by an allergist. Other evaluation methods should also be considered based on the availability of allergist, family preferences, and community comfort levels.

Peanut Consumption

Another question that frequently arises is how often does an infant need to consume peanut after being determined to be peanut tolerant. In the LEAP trial, infants were consuming 2 g of peanut 3 times a week. It is unclear if this amount or this frequency is necessary to maintain tolerance. For many families, this can be challenging, especially if there are other children with peanut allergy in the house or if the infant does not like peanut products.

Because it is unknown if the recommendation of consuming peanut 3 times a week is necessary to maintaining peanut tolerance, it is very important for families of high-risk infants to find a way to maintain peanut in their diet regularly to help ensure they remain tolerant to peanut. In clinical practice, often infants are seen who either passed an OFC to peanut, had negative skin testing to peanut, or safely consumed peanut product at home later develop a peanut allergy. This often occurs after a period of a few weeks without consuming peanut. It is not known if these infants would have developed a peanut allergy had they been regularly consuming peanut. It also is not known the exact frequency with which this happens. However, other studies have documented that people can redevelop a peanut allergy after passing an OFC to peanut when peanut is not regularly ingested.[34]

Timing of Peanut Introduction to Allergy Testing

Another scenario that is frequently encountered is when infants who had negative allergy testing were told to introduce peanut into their diet. Often, when they return for follow-up, they have not yet introduced peanut for a variety of reasons. In these situations, retesting with peanut is recommended because of the risk of resensitization. Although it is unknown how often this occurs in the infant population, other studies have clearly documented resensitization to peanut can occur.[34] In general, the author recommends relying on the peanut SPT for up to 4 weeks. If peanut is not introduced in this window, retesting is recommended.

FUTURE CONSIDERATIONS/SUMMARY

Although unanswered questions, challenges with increasing education, and skepticism about the feasibility of large-scale implementation remain, much is to be gained from adopting new practices that center on early peanut introduction. Recently, much interest has been given to treatment of food allergy. However, prevention can be much more powerful than treatment. When adopted properly, this relatively simple intervention, exposing high-risk infants to peanut early in life, can dramatically decrease the burden of peanut allergy. Caregivers, allergists, and community physicians must work together to develop a system that ensures all infants are being exposed to peanut early in life and high-risk infants are being evaluated by an allergist when needed.

REFERENCES

1. Jackson K, Howie I, Akinbami L. Trends in allergic conditions among children: United States, 1997-2011. National Center for Health Statistics Data Brief; 2013. Available at: www.cdc.gov/nchs/products/databriefs/db121.htm. Accessed December 13, 2016.
2. Avery NJ, King RM, Knight S, et al. Assessment of quality of life in children with peanut allergy. Pediatr Allergy Immunol 2003;14:378–82.
3. King RM, Knibb RC, Hourihane JOB. Impact of peanut allergy on quality of life, stress and anxiety in the family. Allergy 2009;64:461–8.
4. Sampson HA, AcevesS, Bock SA, et al. Food allergy: a practice parameter update-2014. J Allergy Clin Immunol 2014;134:1016–25.
5. American Academy of Pediatrics Committee on Nutrition. Hypoallergenic infant formulas. Pediatrics 2000;106:346–9.
6. National Health and Medical Research Council Infant Feeding Guidelines for Health Workers, 2003. N S W Public Health Bull 2005;16:41.
7. Zeiger RS. Food allergen avoidance in the prevention of food allergy in infants and children. Pediatrics 2003;111:1662–71.
8. Du Toit G, Katz Y, Sasieni P, et al. Early consumption of peanuts in infancy is associated with a low prevalence of peanut allergy. J Allergy Clin Immunol 2008;122: 984–91.
9. Thygarajan A, Burks AW. American Academy of Pediatrics recommendations on the effects of early nutritional interventions on the development of atopic disease. Curr Opin Pediatr 2008;20(6):698–702.
10. Chan ES, Cummings C, Atkinson A, et al. Dietary exposures and allergy prevention in high-risk infants: a joint position statement of the Canadian Society of Allergy and Clinical Immunology and the Canadian Pediatric Society. Allergy Asthma Clin Immunol 2014;10:45.

11. Fleischer DM, Spergel JM, Assaad AH, et al. Primary prevention of allergic disease through nutritional interventions. J Allergy Clin Immunol Pract 2013;1:29–36.

12. Du Toit G, Roberts G, Sayre PH, et al. Randomized trial of peanut consumption in infants at risk for peanut allergy. N Engl J Med 2015;372:803–13.

13. Du Toit G, Sayre PH, Roberts G, et al. Effect of avoidance on peanut allergy after early peanut consumption. N Engl J Med 2016;374:1435–43.

14. Fleischer DM, Sicherer S, Greenhawt, et al. Consensus communication on early peanut introduction and the prevention of peanut allergy in high-risk infants. J Allergy Clin Immunol 2015;136:258–61.

15. Togias A, Cooper SF, Acebal ML, et al. Addendum guidelines for the prevention of peanut allergy in the United States: report of the National Institute of Allergy and Infectious Diseases-sponsored expert panel. J Allergy Clin Immunol 2015; 136:258–61.

16. Osborne NJ, Koplin JJ, Martin PE, et al. Prevalence of challenge-proven IgE-mediated food allergy using population-based sampling and predetermined challenge criteria in infants. J Allergy Clin Immunol 2011;127:668–76.

17. Hourihane JO, Dean TP, Warner JO. Peanut allergy in relation to heredity, maternal diet, and other atopic disease: results of a questionnaire survey, skin prick testing, and food challenges. BMJ 1996;313:518–21.

18. Sicherer SH, Furlong TJ, Maes HH, et al. Genetics of peanut allergy: a twin study. J Allergy Clin Immunol 2000;106:53–6.

19. Liem JJ, Huq S, Kozsyrskyj AL, et al. Should younger siblings of peanut-allergic children be assessed by an allergist before being fed peanut? Allergy Asthma Clin Immunol 2008;4:144–9.

20. Lavine E, Clarke A, Joseph L, et al. Peanut avoidance and peanut allergy diagnosis in siblings of peanut allergic children. Clin Exp Allergy 2015;45:249–54.

21. Gupta RS, Walkner MM, Greenhawt M, et al. Food allergy sensitization and presentation in siblings of food allergic children. J Allergy Clin Immunol 2016;4: 956–62.

22. Madore AM, Vaillancourt VT, Asai Y, et al. HLA-DQB1*02 and DQB1*06:03P are associated with peanut allergy. Eur J Hum Genet 2013;21:1181–4.

23. Levin M, Goga A, Doherty T, et al. Allergy and infant feeding guidelines in the context of resource-constrained settings. J Allergy Clin Immunol 2017;139:455–8.

24. Perkin MR, Logan K, Tseng A, et al. Randomized trial of introduction of allergenic foods in breast-fed infants. N Engl J Med 2016;374:1733–43.

25. Greenhawt M, Chan ES, Fleischer DM, et al. Caregiver and expecting caregiver support for early peanut introduction guidelines. Ann Allergy Asthma Immunol 2018;120:620–5.

26. Abrams EM, Singer AG, Soller L, et al. Knowledge gaps and barriers to early peanut introduction among allergists, pediatricians, and family physicians. J Allergy Clin Immunol Pract 2019;7(2):681–4.

27. Mikhail IJ, Prince B, Stukus D. A quality improvement initiative to increase referrals to an early peanut. Orlando (FL): AAAAI; 2018.

28. Stukus DR, Prince BT, Mikhail I. Implementation of guidelines for early peanut introduction at a pediatric academic center. J Allergy Clin Immunol Pract 2018; 6(5):1784–6.

29. Netting MJ, Campbell DE, Koplin JJ, et al. An Australian consensus on infant feeding guidelines to prevent food allergy: outcomes from the Australian Infant Feeding Summit. J Allergy Clin Immunol Pract 2017;5:1617–24.

30. Assessing the health benefits and risks of the introduction of peanut and hen's egg into the infant diet before 6 months of age in the UK. Available at: https://cot.food.

gov.uk/sites/default/files/jointscncotallergystatementfinal2.pdf. Accessed August 8, 2017.

31. Koplin JJ, Peters RL, Dharmage SC, et al. Understanding the feasibility and implications of implementing early peanut introduction for prevention of peanut allergy. J Allergy Clin Immunol 2016;138:1131–41.

32. Shaker M, Stukus D, Fleischer DM, et al. "To screen or not to screen": comparing the health and economic benefits of early peanut introduction strategies in five countries. Allergy 2018;73(8):1707–14.

33. Tapke DE, Prince BT, Scherzer RS, et al. Implementation of early peanut introduction guidelines among pediatricians. San Francisco (CA): AAAAI; 2019.

34. Fleischer MD, Conover-Walker MK, Christie L, et al. Peanut allergy: recurrence and its management. J Allergy Clin Immunol 2004;114:1195–201.

Managing Younger Siblings of Food Allergic Children

Neha T. Agnihotri, MD[a,1], Dawn K. Lei, MD[a,1], Ruchi S. Gupta, MD, MPH[b],*

KEYWORDS

- Food allergy • Sibling • Children

KEY POINTS

- Current guidelines state that there is insufficient evidence to recommend testing siblings of food allergic children before introduction of potential allergic foods, but the topic remains controversial.
- The prevalence of any clinically reactive food allergy among siblings of food allergic children is noted to be around 13.6%.
- Among siblings of children with food allergy, the rate of sensitization has been shown to be approximately 50%.
- Risk factors, clinical history, and indications for screening must be carefully balanced with the potential for further sensitization, appropriate follow-up, and economic as well as psychosocial impact.
- These measures have implications for nutrition and overall health, home and social interactions, and quality of life.

INTRODUCTION

Food allergies and food-related adverse events have steadily increased in the United States and worldwide. Food avoidance remains one of the mainstays of preventative

Disclosure Statement: Dr. Agnihotri and Dr. Lei have nothing to disclose. Dr. Gupta has reports receiving grants from The National Institute of Health (NIH) (R21 ID # AI135705, R01 ID# AI130348, U01 ID # AI138907), Allergy and Asthma Network, Rho Inc., Stanford Sean N. Parker Center for Allergy Research, Northwestern University Clinical and Translational Sciences Institute (NUCATS), Miller Family Foundation, Aimmune Therapeutics, Mylan Specialty L.P., United-Health Group, Thermo Fisher Scientific, Genentech, and the National Confectioners Association (NCA); is employed by Ann & Robert H. Lurie Children's Hospital of Chicago; is a Professor of Pediatrics at Northwestern University; and serves as a medical consultant/advisor for Before Brands, Pfizer, Kaléo Inc., and DBV Technologies.
^a Department of Medicine, Division of Allergy and Immunology, Northwestern University, 211 E. Ontario, 10th Floor, Suite 1000, Chicago, IL 60611, USA; ^b Institute for Public Health and Medicine, Northwestern University Feinberg School of Medicine, 750 North Lake Shore Drive, Suite #680, Chicago, IL 60611, USA
¹ These authors have equally contributed to this article.
* Corresponding author.
E-mail address: r-gupta@northwestern.edu

Immunol Allergy Clin N Am 39 (2019) 469–480
https://doi.org/10.1016/j.iac.2019.07.001
0889-8561/19/© 2019 Elsevier Inc. All rights reserved.

immunology.theclinics.com

treatment for food allergies. As such, parents of food allergic children strive to maintain a home, school, and social environment that is free of the specified allergen to try to prevent a life-threatening reaction. Consequentially, a common apprehension for families is the likelihood of siblings developing a similar life-threatening food allergy. Current guidelines state that there is insufficient evidence to recommend testing siblings of food allergic children before introduction of potential allergic foods, but the topic continues to remain controversial. Risk factors, clinical history, and indications for screening must be carefully balanced with the potential for further sensitization, appropriate follow-up, and economic as well as psychosocial impact. These measures have implications for nutrition and overall health, home and social interactions, and quality of life.

EPIDEMIOLOGY

The prevalence of food allergies in the population is important to consider when assessing risk, as it informs the growing public health burden and the predictive value of testing. Food allergy affects at least 7.6% of US children (about 1 in 12), with nearly 42% of those children reporting severe, potentially life-threatening allergic reactions and 40% indicating multiple food allergies.[1] Temporal trends in food allergies have been difficult to interpret given the complexity in means of diagnosis.[2] Many studies have relied primarily on self-report although some have included more stringent algorithms, specifically with a double-blind placebo-controlled food challenge. The most common food allergens in the United States that account for most of the food allergic reactions include egg, milk, peanut, tree nuts, wheat, fish, shellfish, and soy.[3]

Most of the studies investigating siblings of food allergic children have focused primarily on peanut allergy alone, reporting an increased risk of peanut allergy in siblings of peanut allergic children.[4–6] A recent large cross-sectional study found that the prevalence of any clinically reactive food allergy among siblings of food allergic children was around 13.6% (or about 1 in 8 children).[7] Among siblings, milk allergy was the most common (5.9%) followed by egg (4.4%) and peanut allergy (3.7%).[7] Milk allergy in siblings was significantly associated with the index child having both an egg and peanut allergy. Index child refers to the child with a confirmed food allergy to whom the sibling comparison is made. Tree nut allergy in the index child was associated with any food allergy in the sibling, particularly sibling egg allergy and sibling peanut allergy. Peanut allergy in the index child did not increase the risk of peanut allergy in their sibling in this particular study.[7]

Along with the rising prevalence of food allergies are the rates of sensitization or the presence of allergen-specific immunoglobulin E (IgE) to food allergens without evidence of clinical symptoms on exposure to those foods. Among siblings of children with food allergy, the rate of sensitization has been shown to be approximately 50%.[7–9] In a study by Gupta and colleagues,[7] wheat sensitization was the most common among allergens (36.5%), followed by milk sensitization (35.4%) and egg sensitization (35.1%). At the same time, nearly one-third of children were neither sensitized nor had any evidence of a clinical food allergy based on history.[7]

Epidemiologic features of food allergy should be taken into consideration when approaching diagnosis and management of food allergies in siblings of food allergic children, recognizing that self-reported food allergy is more common than clinically diagnosed food allergy and rates of sensitization are several folds higher than clinical reactivity.[10]

RISK FACTORS

Food allergy is determined by the interplay of genetic and environmental factors and has a strong association with other atopic diseases. Overall, much remains to be investigated on the risk of food allergy among siblings.

Genetics and Family History

It has been documented that family history is a strong risk factor for food allergy. A large family-based study in the United States found food allergies had significant familial aggregation or the tendency of a disease to cluster in families.[11] This association was significant between food allergic children and their mother as well as their siblings. This study also estimated heritability of the most common food-specific IgE levels, suggesting a range of 0.15 to 0.35.[11] Heritability is a measure that estimates the influence of genetic versus environmental factors on a disease where values closer to one indicate variability in a trait comes from genetic differences.[11] In a small twin study, the concordance rate of peanut allergy among monozygotic twins was much higher than that among dizygotic twins (64.3% vs 6.8%).[12]

Several genome-wide association studies also support a genetic risk for food allergy. A few studies have noted an association between the HLA-DQB1 gene and peanut allergy.[13,14] However, other studies examining the possible relationship between HLA class II alleles and peanut allergy showed no difference between patients with peanut allergy and siblings who are peanut tolerant.[15,16] Similarly, the c11orf30/EMSY locus[17] and SERPINB gene cluster[18] have been identified as genetic risk factors for food allergy. Loss-of-function mutations in the filaggrin gene, which encodes a protein important in the skin's barrier function, have also been found to be a risk factor for IgE-mediated food allergy, independent of atopic dermatitis.[18,19] These genes, however, have not been studied in the context of familial aggregation of food allergies. Moreover, the rate of incidence of food allergies may be rising more quickly than can be accounted for by changes predominantly in the genome sequence.[20]

Environmental Factors

The likelihood of food allergies amongst siblings is additionally guided by shared environmental and lifestyle factors. It is unknown, however, if environmental exposures are more likely to affect those genetically at risk than those without a family history.

Timing of introduction of potentially allergic foods may be a modifiable risk factor for food allergy, although the direct impact among siblings is unclear. Early introduction of potentially allergic foods seems to be associated with a decreased risk in developing food allergy, causing a shift in current consensus guidelines.[10,21,22] More recent literature has shown that delayed oral introduction of foods, such as peanuts, may in fact increase the likelihood of peanut allergy.[22,23] Siblings born after a child was diagnosed with a peanut allergy have been shown to be more likely to never have been exposed to peanuts.[9,24] This may have been influenced by prior recommendations to defer introduction of allergenic foods, although parental anxiety may also contribute based on the older sibling's food allergy history. A large population-based cohort study found that the initial risk of egg allergy in the sibling of a food allergic child was no longer present after controlling for the timing of introduction of egg.[25] The increased risk of egg allergy in the sibling thus was likely related to delayed introduction, in contrast to peanut allergy that may be more guided by genetics, as predicted by heritability estimations.[11,12,25]

Studies have looked at urban and rural lifestyles,[26,27] the presence of pets,[28] and family size and the presence of siblings[29,30] among other associations as predisposing versus protective factors in the development of food allergies. More recent investigation has focused on the role of the microbiome in modifying risk for food allergies, as early childhood seems to be critical for the colonization of the gut by diverse microbiota necessary for oral tolerance.[31] Dietary factors including breastfeeding, probiotics, and vitamin D have additionally been studied.[20] Although literature currently suggests a greater impact on food sensitization than food allergy, environmentally associated evolving patterns and its impact on immune dysregulation continue to be investigated.[32] The relationship of environmental exposures amongst siblings of food allergic children is yet to be well defined.

Association with Other Atopic Conditions

Family history of atopy and the presence of atopic dermatitis are strongly correlated with the development of food sensitization and confirmed food allergy.[3] Having one family member with atopy affects the likelihood of a child having a food allergy, with this risk increasing nearly 2-fold with 2 or more family members.[25] With adjustment for parental atopy and other environmental factors, a history of asthma and eczema was found to be significantly associated with an increased risk for food allergy among siblings.[7] A large population-based study found that in the absence of parental allergic disease, the risk of food allergy was almost doubled among children with atopic siblings.[25] A sibling history of both asthma and allergic rhinitis may predict child egg allergy in particular.[25]

APPROACH TO FOOD ALLERGY TESTING

Evaluation of food allergy begins with a detailed history to identify potential culprit foods and to establish a temporal relationship with acute IgE-mediated symptoms. The low positive predictive value of self-reported symptoms[33] and frequent lack of definitive physical examination findings necessitates additional diagnostic tools.[10,34] Specific IgE (sIgE) testing, which includes skin prick testing (SPT), serum tests, or both, and oral food challenges (OFC) are used to aid in the diagnosis of a food allergy. Testing is traditionally limited only to possible allergens, as a positive sIgE test in the absence of a suggestive clinical history is not sufficient for the diagnosis of a food allergy.

In this light, the proposed evaluation of food allergy in siblings of food allergic patients deviates from the conventional approach. Siblings of food allergic patients frequently present for evaluation of food allergies before exposure to the food of concern. The use of SPT or serum tests in the evaluation of these patients is controversial as the absence of a clinical history of a reaction renders interpretation of these results problematic. Positive sIgE tests may reflect sensitization rather than true food allergy and would necessitate further testing with OFC or risk potential inappropriate diagnosis of food allergy. Furthermore, although threshold values have been developed for several allergenic foods to guide clinicians in their interpretation of these results, the question of whether these same cutoffs can be applied in patients without a history of prior exposure remains less clear.

Skin prick testing, a safe and effective method of detecting sIgE antibodies, has low specificity when applied to food.[10,35] Increasing wheal size is associated with greater clinical relevance of the tested allergen and can be used to predict outcomes of oral food challenges in certain foods.[10,36–39] The positive predictive value of varying wheal sizes reported in other studies depends on the several factors, including the population and food being tested.[10,35] In one pediatric study, for instance, a mean wheal size of 8 mm or greater on peanut SPT had a 95% positive predictive value of positive peanut food challenge.[40] In another study, a wheal size of at least 13 mm was thought to be necessary for diagnosis of food allergy in pediatric patients without prior peanut exposure.[9] Without standardized thresholds for interpretation of SPT results, especially in a population without a history of exposure, SPT should not be used.

Serum-specific IgE testing is another useful tool in the diagnosis of food allergy but similarly requires the context of medical history. Identification of sIgE alone, without a clinical history of reactivity, suggests sensitization to the allergen but not diagnostic of food allergy.[10] Although predictive values for several foods have been established,[41] these values vary based on population, age, and interval since last exposure to allergen, amongst other factors.[10]

Oral food challenge (OFC) can be done in several different ways, including open (or unmasked), single-blinded, double-blinded, and with or without placebo.[42] Double-blind placebo-controlled food challenge is the gold standard for diagnosis of food allergy. All of these procedures are time and labor intensive, which can limit their use.

CURRENT GUIDELINES

In 2010, the National Institute for Allergy and Infectious Disease (NIAID) sponsored expert panel guidelines for food allergy recommended against routine food allergy testing in high-risk children before introduction of allergenic foods such as milk, egg, and peanut.[3] High risk, in this guideline, was defined as a child with a "preexisting severe allergic disease and/or a family history of food allergy."[3] The guidelines did suggest that food allergy evaluation in some populations, such as a sibling with peanut allergy, could be appropriate but argued against routine sIgE.[3]

In 2014, a food allergy practice parameter was released jointly by the AAAAI, ACAAI, and JCAAI. It recommended that in high-risk children, sIgE testing for highly allergenic foods, such as milk, egg, and peanut, could be considered before introduction.[10] High risk in this guideline was defined as the presence of early severe atopic disease or a sibling or parent with peanut allergy.[10]

In 2017, the NIAID addended their peanut allergy prevention guidelines to recommend that caregivers of siblings of peanut allergic children have an informed discussion with their providers regarding the overall benefit versus risk of peanut introduction.

CONSIDERATIONS FOR ROUTINE SCREENING

One reason that routine screening of siblings of food allergic children has been widely debated stems from several studies of siblings of peanut allergic patients. These studies found an increased rate of peanut allergy in siblings of peanut allergic children, ranging from 7% to 8.5%,[4,6,9,12,25] when compared with the rate of peanut allergy in the general population, estimated to be between 1.4% and 3.0%.[6] Another study demonstrated that the risk of an IgE-mediated reaction to peanuts in siblings of peanut allergic children was 5.2%, with 5 of the 8 reactions presenting as anaphylaxis.[6] It is likely that the specific inclusion of siblings with peanut allergy as a risk factor for food allergy in the 2014 practice parameter update comes from consideration of these studies.

Parental anxiety about food introduction following an allergic reaction in another child may be another reason that families seek food allergy testing. Ninety three percent of parents in one study reported that their first child's food allergy affected the introduction of foods to younger siblings, with 54% delaying certain foods and 64% of parents avoiding introduction of certain foods.[43] A significant percentage of parents (82%) reported anxiety when introducing foods to the younger child.[43] Interestingly, 82% of parents in another study reported that they would not follow clinician advice for at-home introduction without testing.[6] A proportion of these parents may hesitate to introduce certain foods due to the difficulty of safely feeding an allergenic food to one child without also exposing their allergic sibling. In these families, providing teaching about methods to safely introduce to one sibling may be necessary to facilitate home introduction. Given the risks that delayed food introduction may have on the development of food allergy,[22] discussion of screening tests before home introduction versus in-office supervised introduction may be warranted. However, physicians should note that a proportion of parents would still choose not to introduce certain foods at home despite negative testing. As shown by Begin and colleagues,[6] 15% of parents did not introduce peanut into their child's diet and 34% did not regularly introduce (less than monthly consumption) peanut despite negative peanut food allergy evaluation.

Children with other food allergy risk factors, in addition to a sibling with food allergy, should be referred to a specialist for evaluation of food allergies. The decision to undergo testing before certain food introduction can then be made on an individual basis after frank discussion between the provider and family about the risks and benefits of screening.

CONSIDERATIONS AGAINST ROUTINE SCREENING

In addition to the poor predictive value of sIgE testing,[3,7] several other concerns argue against routine screening of siblings of food allergic patients. Foremost against routine screening is the high rate of asymptomatic food sensitization without true allergy, which has been estimated to range from 30% to 50% in the general population.[4,8,44,45] One study found that 22% of children with positive SPT to peanuts were sensitized but not allergic and were able to consume peanuts without difficulty.[4] Gupta and colleagues[7] showed that 53% of siblings of food allergic children (or 1 out of every 2 tested) were sensitized but not clinically food allergic. Comparatively, only 13.6% of siblings in this study had a true food allergy.[7]

With such high rates of asymptomatic sensitization, many children may be misdiagnosed with food allergy and recommended inappropriate food avoidance.[7] Some physicians or providers may incorrectly interpret positive sIgE testing as diagnostic of food allergy and fail to refer these children to allergy specialists for additional evaluation and confirmatory testing, instead opting to advise continued avoidance of tested foods. Similarly, some parents may come to assume that positive testing confirms food allergy and decline to seek or complete further testing. For some children, if sIgE testing results in values greater than certain cutoff levels, they may be deemed allergic and may never be offered the opportunity to undergo an OFC, despite the fact that some percentage may be found to tolerate the food in question.[46] Indeed, 3.4% of cases of peanut allergy have been estimated to result from overdiagnosis by SPT screening.[46]

The finding of positive sIgE testing warrants further assessment to confirm or refute the diagnosis of food allergy, often done through an oral food challenge.[6] However, OFCs are frequently delayed, with one study demonstrating that 54% of OFCs were postponed by greater than 12 months after sIgE levels became less than 2kUA/L, a value associated with a high likelihood of passing an oral challenge.[47] In that study, the average time to OFC was 35.5 months in the delayed group and more than 4 months in the nondelayed group.[47]

A multitude of explanations may be given for deferring OFCs, both from the family/caregiver and from the clinician. Potential reasons may include lack of resources (time, staff, space, training), poor reimbursement, and concern for a potential reaction.[47,48] For foods without well-defined cutoff levels or component-resolved diagnostics to guide probability of oral tolerance, persistently positive sIgE test results may also delay OFCs. Age of the child may also be a cause of delay as some providers or caregivers may perceive that the child will not cooperate with an OFC or may not be able to express the development of symptoms.[42,47] Several studies, including LEAP[22] and HealthNuts[49] have demonstrated that OFC in young children is both feasible and safe. For others, the presence of positive sIgE testing may cause many families to defer evaluation with OFC due to concern for development of reaction and instead proceed with avoidance of those selected foods.[7] This apprehension is particularly pervasive in families who already have a food allergic child.

Regardless of reason, any unnecessary delay in food introduction may potentially increase the risk of true food allergy development of the avoided food, as has recently been shown by the protective effect of early introduction of peanuts.[22]

ECONOMIC IMPACT

Screening siblings of food allergic children has significant implications for economic cost and burden. Although there is no study that has directly calculated the cost of implementation of routine screening of siblings of food allergic children, studies have been completed to evaluate the cost of food allergy and screening before early peanut introduction.

Shaker and colleagues[46] examined the cost and outcomes of 2 different approaches to early peanut introduction. They compared a no-screening approach to early peanut introduction against screening peanut skin testing and in-office peanut introduction in high-risk infants. Not only did the no-screening approach demonstrate superior clinical outcomes in terms of the number of peanut allergy cases prevented but it also demonstrated significant economic benefits. Compared with the no-screening approach, the cost to prevent one peanut-allergic reaction in the high-risk cohort was $20,393 using SPT or $71,020 using sIgE. In their cost calculations, they found that screening the 16% of the infant population with early onset eczema and/ or egg allergy in the United States (approximately 641,522 infants) before peanut introduction would levy an additional cost of $654 million.

Recent US Census records suggest that there are currently approximately 73.8 million children in the United States.[50] Approximately 1.0% to 2.1% of the pediatric population is composed of younger siblings of peanut allergic children.[6,9] The implementation of routine screening of these approximately 730,000 to 1.5 million siblings of peanut allergic children, which does not account for the larger population of siblings of any food allergic child, would render a substantial financial burden.

Furthermore, the cost of the consequences of screening cannot be neglected. As discussed earlier, screening may identify a large number of patients with asymptomatic sensitization and result in misdiagnosis of food allergy. The annual medical cost of food allergy has been estimated at $4184 per year per child.[51] Although patient care and outcomes remain the priority, the economic impact of managing siblings of food allergic patients must also be considered.

EFFECT ON NUTRITIONAL INTAKE AND GROWTH

Health considerations should be emphasized when deciding on an approach to siblings of food allergic children. Food restriction may occur due to family avoidance of the food allergic child's allergens or due to presumed diagnosis or misdiagnosis of food allergy in the sibling. However, limiting dietary intake can have a direct impact on the essential nutrients a child receives and thereby his/her growth and development. For instance, milk avoidance can reduce daily required intake of calcium and vitamin D, potentially affecting bone mineral status as well as motor development.[52] Wheat, which provides complex carbohydrates, is one of the primary sources of energy for the brain.[53] Milk, egg, and soy are important sources of protein and fat, which fuel energy and growth.[53]

Growth serves as a strong surrogate marker for assessing adequate overall energy and protein intake in children. Indeed, children with 2 or more food allergies are often smaller, by weight and particularly by height, for their age.[54,55] In addition, Kwashiorkor, a nutritional disorder due to severe protein malnutrition, has been reported in children in the United States on allergen elimination diets.[56] It is therefore important to address the unintended health impacts that may occur due to restriction of foods for siblings of food allergic children where there is not a clinical need. In addition to children with food allergies, siblings avoiding certain foods for any reason should receive an annual nutrition assessment to incorporate alternative nutrient-dense foods into the diet and prevent growth impairment or inadequate nutritional intake.[55]

PSYCHOSOCIAL IMPACT

Quality of life for the family is an important consideration when approaching management of siblings of food allergic children. Food allergy has been associated with negative psychosocial impact and poorer quality of life for children with food allergy and their families. As such, when managing siblings of food allergic children, extrapolating a food allergy for the younger child may have psychosocial repercussions that can hinder emotional and mental well-being. For instance, children may experience teasing or isolation in social settings because of their presumed food allergy. The stress surrounding the navigation of food avoidance or social interactions can progress to states of anxiety or depression.[57–59]

Fear of adverse events and anxiety about eating is central to concerns surrounding food allergies and may be more acutely perceived by parents than the child.[60,61] Food allergy has a significant effect on daily family life such as a meal preparation and family social activities.[62] Many parents may prefer minimizing the risk and anxiety of possible exposure by avoiding certain activities all together and creating a consistent environment in the home, which could consequentially affect siblings of food allergic children.[62] In addition to anxiety, time and financial constraints may also dictate meal preparation and thus siblings may end up adopting similar dietary patterns as the food allergic child. The fear of a potential reaction and the disruption due to measures taken to avoid allergen exposure have been shown to be factors associated with a lower quality of life, rather than the actual clinical reactivity experienced by food intake.[63]

More literature is emerging that investigates the role of parental anxiety after having a previous child with an allergy and how that influences the decision to introduce potentially allergenic foods.[9] A study of peanut introduction in younger siblings of peanut allergic children examined levels of anxiety related to peanut introduction.[6] Parents were more likely to introduce at home after negative testing and had increased apprehension to do so without any testing. It is unclear that the fear is based on actual risk but rather seems to be more likely influenced by the negative experiences with the older sibling's allergy.[6] For patients found to be peanut tolerant who were followed-up after a year, the main reported reason for not introducing the tolerated food, even at low frequency, was difficulty managing risk of cross-contamination or contact with the older sibling.[6] Of note, for a significant portion of patients who reintroduced peanut at home, there was no cited accidental contact with the allergic sibling.[6] Some strategies suggested for introduction of foods to the younger sibling that the older child was allergic to, designating a space in the house for consumption, dedicating a time in the week when the older child was absent, and eating only outside the household at restaurants or at other family members' homes.

Ultimately, psychosocial concerns remain an integral part of food allergy management and anticipatory guidance. Physicians should remain alert as well about families' hesitations and be willing to offer more guidance and support to this effect.

SUMMARY

Although the proportion of siblings who are sensitized to a food without clinical reactivity is high in comparison to those with a true food allergy, there is still a known increased risk amongst siblings of children with food allergies that has led to much apprehension and controversy about management. The appropriateness of testing and further steps for management of sensitization in the absence of history of clinical reactivity should be discussed with parents. These siblings are likely to be mislabeled as food allergic when they are in fact tolerant to the food.[7] This has implications for children down the road, including increased risk of developing allergy due to avoidance, potential for growth and development restrictions, and a negative impact on quality of life.

REFERENCES

1. Gupta RS, Warren CM, Smith BM, et al. The public health impact of parent-reported childhood food allergies in the United States. Pediatrics 2018;142(6) [pii:e20181235].
2. Ben-Shoshan M, Turnbull E, Clarke A. Food allergy: temporal trends and determinants. Curr Allergy Asthma Rep 2012;12(4):346–72.
3. Boyce JA, Assa'ad A, Burks AW, et al. Guidelines for the diagnosis and management of food allergy in the United States: summary of the NIAID-sponsored expert panel report. J Allergy Clin Immunol 2010;126(6):1105–18.
4. Liem JJ, Huq S, Kozyrskyj AL, et al. Should younger siblings of peanut-allergic children be assessed by an allergist before being fed peanut? Allergy Asthma Clin Immunol 2008;4(4):144–9.
5. Hourihane JO, Dean TP, Warner JO. Peanut allergy in relation to heredity, maternal diet, and other atopic diseases: results of a questionnaire survey, skin prick testing, and food challenges. BMJ 1996;313(7056):518–21.
6. Begin P, Graham F, Killer K, et al. Introduction of peanuts in younger siblings of children with peanut allergy: a prospective, double-blinded assessment of risk, of diagnostic tests, and an analysis of patient preferences. Allergy 2016; 71(12):1762–71.
7. Gupta RS, Walkner MM, Greenhawt M, et al. Food allergy sensitization and presentation in siblings of food allergic children. J Allergy Clin Immunol Pract 2016; 4(5):956–62.
8. Rance F, Juchet A, Bremont F, et al. Correlations between skin prick tests using commercial extracts and fresh foods, specific IgE, and food challenges. Allergy 1997;52(10):1031–5.
9. Lavine E, Clarke A, Joseph L, et al. Peanut avoidance and peanut allergy diagnosis in siblings of peanut allergic children. Clin Exp Allergy 2015;45(1):249–54.
10. Sampson HA, Aceves S, Bock SA, et al. Food allergy: a practice parameter update-2014. J Allergy Clin Immunol 2014;134(5):1016–25.e43.
11. Tsai HJ, Kumar R, Pongracic J, et al. Familial aggregation of food allergy and sensitization to food allergens: a family-based study. Clin Exp Allergy 2009; 39(1):101–9.
12. Sicherer SH, Furlong TJ, Maes HH, et al. Genetics of peanut allergy: a twin study. J Allergy Clin Immunol 2000;106(1 Pt 1):53–6.
13. Madore AM, Vaillancourt VT, Asai Y, et al. HLA-DQB1*02 and DQB1*06:03P are associated with peanut allergy. Eur J Hum Genet 2013;21(10):1181–4.

14. Hong X, Hao K, Ladd-Acosta C, et al. Genome-wide association study identifies peanut allergy-specific loci and evidence of epigenetic mediation in US children. Nat Commun 2015;6:6304.

15. Howell WM, Turner SJ, Hourihane JO, et al. HLA class II DRB1, DQB1 and DPB1 genotypic associations with peanut allergy: evidence from a family-based and case-control study. Clin Exp Allergy 1998;28(2):156–62.

16. Dreskin SC, Tripputi MT, Aubrey MT, et al. Peanut-allergic subjects and their peanut-tolerant siblings have large differences in peanut-specific IgG that are independent of HLA class II. Clin Immunol 2010;137(3):366–73.

17. Asai Y, Eslami A, van Ginkel CD, et al. Genome-wide association study and meta-analysis in multiple populations identifies new loci for peanut allergy and establishes C11orf30/EMSY as a genetic risk factor for food allergy. J Allergy Clin Immunol 2018;141(3):991–1001.

18. Marenholz I, Grosche S, Kalb B, et al. Genome-wide association study identifies the SERPINB gene cluster as a susceptibility locus for food allergy. Nat Commun 2017;8(1):1056.

19. Brown SJ, Asai Y, Cordell HJ, et al. Loss-of-function variants in the filaggrin gene are a significant risk factor for peanut allergy. J Allergy Clin Immunol 2011;127(3): 661–7.

20. Tan TH, Ellis JA, Saffery R, et al. The role of genetics and environment in the rise of childhood food allergy. Clin Exp Allergy 2012;42(1):20–9.

21. Chan ES, Abrams EM, Hildebrand KJ, et al. Early introduction of foods to prevent food allergy. Allergy Asthma Clin Immunol 2018;14(Suppl 2):57.

22. Du Toit G, Roberts G, Sayre PH, et al. Randomized trial of peanut consumption in infants at risk for peanut allergy. N Engl J Med 2015;372(9):803–13.

23. Du Toit G, Sayre PH, Roberts G, et al. Effect of avoidance on peanut allergy after early peanut consumption. N Engl J Med 2016;374(15):1435–43.

24. Ben-Shoshan M, Kagan RS, Alizadehfar R, et al. Is the prevalence of peanut allergy increasing? A 5-year follow-up study in children in Montreal. J Allergy Clin Immunol 2009;123(4):783–8.

25. Koplin JJ, Allen KJ, Gurrin LC, et al. The impact of family history of allergy on risk of food allergy: a population-based study of infants. Int J Environ Res Public Health 2013;10(11):5364–77.

26. Alfven T, Braun-Fahrlander C, Brunekreef B, et al. Allergic diseases and atopic sensitization in children related to farming and anthroposophic lifestyle–the PARSIFAL study. Allergy 2006;61(4):414–21.

27. Liu AH. Revisiting the hygiene hypothesis for allergy and asthma. J Allergy Clin Immunol 2015;136(4):860–5.

28. Ownby DR, Johnson CC, Peterson EL. Exposure to dogs and cats in the first year of life and risk of allergic sensitization at 6 to 7 years of age. JAMA 2002;288(8): 963–72.

29. Jarvis D, Chinn S, Luczynska C, et al. The association of family size with atopy and atopic disease. Clin Exp Allergy 1997;27(3):240–5.

30. Mattes J, Karmaus W, Moseler M, et al. Accumulation of atopic disorders within families: a sibling effect only in the offspring of atopic fathers. Clin Exp Allergy 1998;28(12):1480–6.

31. Ho HE, Bunyavanich S. Role of the microbiome in food allergy. Curr Allergy Asthma Rep 2018;18(4):27.

32. Yu JE, Mallapaty A, Miller RL. It's not just the food you eat: environmental factors in the development of food allergies. Environ Res 2018;165:118–24.

33. Rona RJ, Keil T, Summers C, et al. The prevalence of food allergy: a meta-analysis. J Allergy Clin Immunol 2007;120(3):638–46.
34. Sampson HA. Food allergy. Part 2: diagnosis and management. J Allergy Clin Immunol 1999;103(6):981–9.
35. Sampson HA. Comparative study of commercial food antigen extracts for the diagnosis of food hypersensitivity. J Allergy Clin Immunol 1988;82(5 Pt 1):718–26.
36. Sporik R, Hill DJ, Hosking CS. Specificity of allergen skin testing in predicting positive open food challenges to milk, egg and peanut in children. Clin Exp Allergy 2000;30(11):1540–6.
37. Verstege A, Mehl A, Rolinck-Werninghaus C, et al. The predictive value of the skin prick test weal size for the outcome of oral food challenges. Clin Exp Allergy 2005;35(9):1220–6.
38. Pucar F, Kagan R, Lim H, et al. Peanut challenge: a retrospective study of 140 patients. Clin Exp Allergy 2001;31(1):40–6.
39. Saarinen KM, Suomalainen H, Savilahti E. Diagnostic value of skin-prick and patch tests and serum eosinophil cationic protein and cow's milk-specific IgE in infants with cow's milk allergy. Clin Exp Allergy 2001;31(3):423–9.
40. Roberts G, Lack G. Diagnosing peanut allergy with skin prick and specific IgE testing. J Allergy Clin Immunol 2005;115(6):1291–6.
41. Sampson HA. Utility of food-specific IgE concentrations in predicting symptomatic food allergy. J Allergy Clin Immunol 2001;107(5):891–6.
42. Nowak-Wegrzyn A, Assa'ad AH, Bahna SL, et al. Work group report: oral food challenge testing. J Allergy Clin Immunol 2009;123(6 Suppl):S365–83.
43. McHenry M, Watson W. Impact of primary food allergies on the introduction of other foods amongst Canadian children and their siblings. Allergy Asthma Clin Immunol 2014;10(1):26.
44. Bock SA, Atkins FM. Patterns of food hypersensitivity during sixteen years of double-blind, placebo-controlled food challenges. J Pediatr 1990;117(4):561–7.
45. Sampson HA, Albergo R. Comparison of results of skin tests, RAST, and double-blind, placebo-controlled food challenges in children with atopic dermatitis. J Allergy Clin Immunol 1984;74(1):26–33.
46. Shaker M, Stukus D, Chan ES, et al. "To screen or not to screen": comparing the health and economic benefits of early peanut introduction strategies in five countries. Allergy 2018;73(8):1707–14.
47. Couch C, Franxman T, Greenhawt M. The economic effect and outcome of delaying oral food challenges. Ann Allergy Asthma Immunol 2016;116(5):420–4.
48. Pongracic JA, Bock SA, Sicherer SH. Oral food challenge practices among allergists in the United States. J Allergy Clin Immunol 2012;129(2):564–6.
49. Koplin JJ, Wake M, Dharmage SC, et al. Cohort profile: The HealthNuts Study: population prevalence and environmental/genetic predictors of food allergy. Int J Epidemiol 2015;44(4):1161–71.
50. Child population: number of children (in millions) ages 0–17 in the United States by age, 1950–2017 and projected 2018–2050. Available at: https://www.childstats.gov/americaschildren/tables/pop1.asp. Accessed January 24, 2019.
51. Gupta R, Holdford D, Bilaver L, et al. The economic impact of childhood food allergy in the United States. JAMA Pediatr 2013;167(11):1026–31.
52. Jensen VB, Jorgensen IM, Rasmussen KB, et al. Bone mineral status in children with cow milk allergy. Pediatr Allergy Immunol 2004;15(6):562–5.
53. Mehta H, Groetch M, Wang J. Growth and nutritional concerns in children with food allergy. Curr Opin Allergy Clin Immunol 2013;13(3):275–9.

54. Flammarion S, Santos C, Guimber D, et al. Diet and nutritional status of children with food allergies. Pediatr Allergy Immunol 2011;22(2):161–5.
55. Christie L, Hine RJ, Parker JG, et al. Food allergies in children affect nutrient intake and growth. J Am Diet Assoc 2002;102(11):1648–51.
56. Liu T, Howard RM, Mancini AJ, et al. Kwashiorkor in the United States: fad diets, perceived and true milk allergy, and nutritional ignorance. Arch Dermatol 2001; 137(5):630–6.
57. Cummings AJ, Knibb RC, King RM, et al. The psychosocial impact of food allergy and food hypersensitivity in children, adolescents and their families: a review. Allergy 2010;65(8):933–45.
58. Lyons AC, Forde EM. Food allergy in young adults: perceptions and psychological effects. J Health Psychol 2004;9(4):497–504.
59. Patten SB, Williams JV. Self-reported allergies and their relationship to several Axis I disorders in a community sample. Int J Psychiatry Med 2007;37(1):11–22.
60. Sicherer SH, Noone SA, Munoz-Furlong A. The impact of childhood food allergy on quality of life. Ann Allergy Asthma Immunol 2001;87(6):461–4.
61. King RM, Knibb RC, Hourihane JO. Impact of peanut allergy on quality of life, stress and anxiety in the family. Allergy 2009;64(3):461–8.
62. Bollinger ME, Dahlquist LM, Mudd K, et al. The impact of food allergy on the daily activities of children and their families. Ann Allergy Asthma Immunol 2006;96(3): 415–21.
63. Marklund B, Ahlstedt S, Nordstrom G. Health-related quality of life in food hypersensitive schoolchildren and their families: parents' perceptions. Health Qual Life Outcomes 2006;4:48.

Oral Food Challenges in Infants and Toddlers

Justin Greiwe, MD[a,b,*]

KEYWORDS

• Food allergy • Oral food challenge • Anaphylaxis • Infants • Epinephrine

KEY POINTS

- Oral food challenges are a critical procedure to identify patients with IgE-mediated food allergy when the history and testing are not specific enough to confirm a diagnosis.
- Food challenges in infants and toddlers are both safe and practical in a clinical setting.
- Comprehensive past medical history is critical in the diagnosis of food allergy and should be used to determine subsequent testing and interpretation of results.
- Food allergies are associated with significant social and psychological consequences that often are overlooked by health care professionals.
- More emphasis needs to be placed on food challenge education and hands-on experience during fellowship training.

INTRODUCTION

Oral food challenges (OFCs) remain the gold standard for diagnosis of food allergy. Although double-blind placebo-controlled OFCs are the criteria standard, they are time consuming and unrealistic in a clinical setting and, therefore, reserved mainly for research purposes. Open (nonblinded) challenges are the method of choice, with ingestion of meal-sized portions of the concerning food prepared in its usual state. OFCs often are recommended when there is an approximately 50% likelihood that the food challenged will be tolerated based on available data and clinical history.

SAFETY

OFCs are an indispensable tool for accurately diagnosing clinically relevant food allergy; however, their use in clinical practice is not widespread due in part to supposed safety concerns. Infants especially are perceived as high-risk because they are

Disclosure: Dr J. Greiwe is a speaker for Regeneron and Sanofi Genzyme and on advisory boards for AstraZeneca and Genentech.
[a] Bernstein Allergy Group Inc, 8444 Winton Road, Cincinnati, OH 45231, USA; [b] Division of Immunology/Allergy Section, Department of Internal Medicine, The University of Cincinnati College of Medicine, Cincinnati, OH, USA
* 8444 Winton Road, Cincinnati, OH 45231.
E-mail address: jcgreiwe@gmail.com

smaller, nonverbal, and more difficult to objectively monitor. Allergic reactions in this age group present diagnostic challenges that can dissuade caregivers from providing OFCs for their patients. Infants, for example, are unable to describe certain symptoms, such as pruritus or throat tightness, and can develop behavioral changes and increased irritability that can be difficult to interpret because they may occur in healthy infants as well. Objective pulmonary function testing is also not feasible in this age group, so an accurate assessment of lung function is not available. With time and experience, recognizing subtle, nonverbal infant cues of a reaction becomes easier and can include signs like ear picking, tongue rubbing, neck scratching, putting a hand in the mouth, and a change in general demeanor (ie, quiet, withdrawn, clingy, or fussy).[1] Differentiating between normal, immunoglobulin E (IgE)-mediated, and non–IgE-mediated symptoms is where physician experience comes into play.

Despite perceived concerns, the data suggest OFCs, including infant OFCs, are both safe and practical in a clinical setting.[2–5] Akuete and colleagues,[6] for example, analyzed 6377 OFCs from 2008 to 2013 and a large majority (86%) were challenged without a reaction. Only 2% required epinephrine, leaving 98% of OFCs completed without symptoms of anaphylaxis, demonstrating OFCs are much safer than previously thought. This is in stark contrast to previous studies where epinephrine usage during OFCs was closer to 6% to 33%.[7–11] Late-phase and biphasic reactions after OFCs are rare, with an estimated occurrence of approximately 1.5% to 4% in previously published studies.[12–14] One known fatality has been documented (2017) since the description of modern OFCs published in 1976.[15] Additional data demonstrate safety and efficacy in children less than 18 months old as well, with most reactions being mild in presentation and limited to the skin. Infants seem to have a low rate of anaphylaxis with infrequent use of epinephrine and intensive care unit admissions.[2–4,16–18]

ACCURACY OF TESTING

Accurately interpreting serum and skin testing for food allergies has been an ongoing issue in the field of allergy and immunology, often leading to mislabeling of the food allergy diagnosis. This discrepancy is due in part to both the poor sensitivity and specificity of current testing available as well as the impressive differences in user interpretation. Practice approaches involving testing administration and interpretation vary greatly within the subspecialty, which has likely led to a misrepresentation of true IgE-mediated food allergy versus sensitization. Both skin prick testing (SPT) and food–serum-specific IgE (sIgE) testing are relied on heavily to screen patients for sensitivity to specific foods and to determine if OFCs should be considered. SPT to foods has a high negative predictive value (NPV) but poor positive predictive value (PPV) of only 50%.[18] Negative SPT effectively confirms the absence of an IgE-mediated process (NPV >95%).[19] Skin testing protocols, extracts, and testing devices may vary, which can affect reliability of testing. ImmunoCAP is the most common serologic method used to test for food allergies; however, alternative assays are not identical.

Past medical history, therefore, is critical in the diagnosis of food allergy and should be used to determine subsequent testing and interpretation of results. Many patients come to an office with positive testing but no history of ingestion or reaction. The most common example is an infant with moderate/severe eczema who underwent broad-panel sIgE food testing. Age, clinical history, and history of sensitivity but no exposure also may affect accuracy of testing. To make matters more confusing, a large proportion of patients have intermediate values on skin and/or serum testing.

Criteria indicating high or low probability of passing vary among studies but there are certain trends that improve the accuracy of testing. Larger SPT wheal size (>8 mm) and higher food-sIgE levels are associated with persistent food allergy and higher rates of failed challenges. Rate of change of these levels can help predict likelihood that food allergy has resolved.[20,21] There have been multiple attempts to provide guidance based on sIgE levels associated with a 50% PPV and 95% PPV for clinical allergy.[22,23] Guidelines suggest using the 50% PPV to guide the timing of an OFC. The Standardized Clinical Assessment and Management Plan for food challenges is another tool that has been published that attempts to improve sIgE and SPT thresholds and triage patients safely into either a low-intensity or high-intensity care setting for OFC.[24] Although these values can act as a guide, serum testing should always be interpreted on a case-by-case basis. Factors such as an absence of history of a clinical reaction to the food, a prior history tolerance to a food, African American race, concomitant inhalant allergies, atopic dermatitis (AD), older age, and high total IgE can all lower the probability of a true clinical food allergy. Fleischer et al. examined a cohort of 125 AD patients and reported that no patient with a sIgE level below the 95% predictive decision point for milk, egg, or peanut failed an OFC suggesting that reliance on serum food-specific IgE testing to determine the need for food elimination diets in children, especially those with AD, is not sufficient.[6] In addition, Frischmeyer-Guerrerio et al. estimated that AD subjects with a milk IgE of 43 kUA/L, egg IgE of 28 kUA/L, and peanut IgE of 34 kUA/L had at least a 50% chance of not being allergic to the food.[25] Relying solely on these predictive values to make clinical decisions can lead to misdiagnosis, as demonstrated in the clinical scenario outlined in **Table 1**.

According to the available data, the 3-year-old boy described in **Table 1** should not have been challenged to any of these foods. Instead of condemning this patient to years of restrictive eating and social isolation, an honest conversation was started with the parents on the risks and benefits of attempting OFCs under observation in a supervised setting. Although this conversation is often difficult for all parties involved, it is necessary to provide the best possible care for patients. Although the example provided in **Table 1** is an extreme case, there are millions of children in the United States avoiding foods that they might not be allergic to, subjecting families to increased financial burdens (clinician visits, specialty foods and diets, and lost

---

Table 1
Exception to the rule, a recurring theme with oral food challenges

A 3-year-old boy with a history of multiple food allergies and severe eczema as an infant comes to your office for further evaluation. At 12 months old the patient had broad-panel food sIgE completed which showed the following:

Total IgE 3873 IU/mL	Sesame 87.6 kU/L	Almond 64.1 kU/L
Egg white 75.3 kU/L	Wheat >100 kU/L	Cashew >100 kU/L
Cow's milk >100 kU/L	Chickpea >100 kU/L	Pistachio 97.5 kU/L
Pea >100 kU/L	Lentils 96.1 kU/L	Walnut 30.8 kU/L
Hazelnut 68.6 kU/L	Pecan 10.2 kU/L	

- SPT: wheals anywhere from 6 mm to 9 mm; some skin tests were negative.
- Told to avoid all these foods despite never ingesting leading to a very restrictive diet, poor growth, and poor nutrition.
- Eczema has significantly improved over the last 2 years and recent SPT demonstrate wheals anywhere from 6 mm to 9 mm; some skin tests were negative.
- Passed OFC: baked then uncooked eggs, baked milk, all tree nuts except cashew/pistachio, chickpea, pea, lentils, and sesame.
- Failed OFC: wheat (with final dose) and cashew/pistachio.

productivity due to time off work/school), nutritional deficiencies/lifetime of picky eating, sibling effects (entire family often practices avoidance even if they do not have a food allergy), and social/psychological consequences. To avoid accidental exposures, some parents try to control all situations, leading to isolation and fear. Hypervigilance can instill excessive amounts of anxiety in food-allergic children, which sometimes spills over into other areas of life, leading some parents to home-school, forbid normal social interaction like sleepovers and birthday parties, and even avoid traveling on airplanes or sporting events.

To save parents and patients from going down this rabbit hole of fear and anxiety, physicians must take it upon themselves to properly educate families of food allergic children on the real risks of accidental exposure and challenge those whose history and evaluation might not be consistent with an IgE-mediated response. The example discussed previously suggests that current testing modalities are inaccurate and should be approached with more skepticism rather than thought of as absolute truth. Good old-fashioned comprehensive food allergy history and clinical judgment are still important when diagnosing food allergy, and blind reliance on testing has led to a lot of misdiagnosis.

Food testing that is not validated includes food-specific IgG and IgG4 tests, which typically yield multiple positive results, leading to unnecessary avoidance and restrictive diets. Positive results with these tests likely represent normal immune responses to foods and should not be used to diagnose food allergy or food intolerance. Other tests that should be avoided include sublingual or intracutaneous provocation tests, tests of lymphocyte activation, kinesiology, cytotoxic tests, and electrodermal testing.

Food allergy diagnosis and testing are still as much art as science and remain an area of medicine where experience and clinical judgment still matter. To help improve the accuracy of food testing, several additional methods are being investigated to aid in diagnosis and monitoring for tolerance. These include IgE epitope specificity, component-resolved diagnostics, IgE/IgG4 ratio, cellular-based assays, basophil activation test, and specific IgA and IgA2 levels.[22,26–32] Ultimately, current modalities are inadequate, and both skin and serum testing have limited predictive power to determine which patients are likely to pass an OFC.[33–35] More sensitive and specific biomarkers are needed that provide better correlation with clinical reactivity to both specific IgE-mediated and non–IgE-mediated food reactions.

THE NUTS AND BOLTS OF FOOD CHALLENGES

The approach to OFCs should be straightforward and handled with the same attention to detail as with other risky procedures done in the office setting like subcutaneous allergen immunotherapy or drug challenges. All OFCs should be standardized and follow these simple steps:

1. Initial assessment, including physical examination
2. Monitoring of vital signs before, during, and after challenge
3. Administration of food in a standardized manner: starting low and gradually increasing until a cumulative dose equivalent to a standard portion for age is consumed
4. Symptoms (if present) treated

This pattern should be repeated in a similar manner for all patients, mirroring an assembly line to maximize efficiency and minimize errors. There should be predetermined protocols that include both high-risk and low-risk protocols depending on the clinical history of reaction as well as results of serum and/or skin testing (**Table 2**).[36]

Table 2
Risk assessment for oral food challenges

Low risk of reaction	1. Recent accidental ingestion to small amount of food without clinical symptoms
	2. Favorable test results[b]
High risk of reaction	1. Recent reaction to the food in the past 6–12 mo
	2. Diagnostic or high-positive test results
Low risk of severe reaction[a]	1. No past severe reactions
	2. Food not usually implicated in severe food-induced anaphylaxis (eg, meat, fruit, and vegetable[c])
	3. No asthma
High risk of severe reaction	1. Past severe reaction
	2. Severe reaction to trace amounts of food
	3. Food frequently implicated in fatal and near-fatal food-induced anaphylaxis (eg, peanut, tree nuts, fish, shellfish, and seeds)
	4. Asthma (regardless of severity)
	5. Conditions that may affect the resuscitation: cardiovascular disease, difficult vascular access or intubation, β-blocker medication

[a] Severe reaction is defined as any lower respiratory or cardiovascular symptoms or any 4 organ systems involved.
[b] Laboratory cutpoints for deferring OFC were defined for a few foods in children. These cutpoints have not been evaluated in adults with food allergy.
[c] A food is capable of inducing a severe anaphylactic reaction, including fruits and vegetables. The patient's previous reactions should be a guide for assessing the risk of a potential reaction during an OFC.
Adapted from Nowak-Wegrzyn A, Assa'ad AH, Bahna SL, et al. Work Group report: oral food challenge testing. J Allergy Clin Immunol 2009;123(6 Suppl):S367; with permission.

For food challenges in a clinical setting to be successful, the office needs to be set up for success. This includes maximizing efficiency of the physical layout of the office as well as the supporting staff. Key components to performing successful food challenges are outlined in **Fig. 1**.

Although not everyone is able to change the layout of an office due to space limitations and/or cost, there are certain office setups that are better suited for providing multiple food challenges at once. A large common dosing area that is clearly visible from the nursing station offers many advantages, including

1. Quick, easy dosing administration
2. The ability to clearly observe clinical reactions
3. More nurses available to administer doses and check vital signs/peak flow
4. Allowing multiple challenges to be performed at once

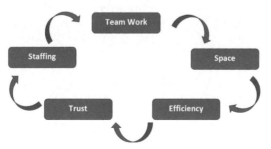

Fig. 1. Key components to performing successful food challenges in clinical practice.

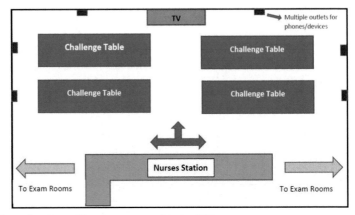

Fig. 2. Example of an office space amenable to OFCs.

5. Not monopolizing examination rooms; providing a community feel, fostering healthy patient-patient and parent-parent interactions
6. Added benefit of increasing distractions for kids undergoing challenges

An example of an ideal setup is included in **Fig. 2**. In this setup, there is a clear line of vision from the nurses station to the challenge tables, with a room large enough to perform multiple challenges and skin tests at the same time. Patients experiencing more severe reactions can be removed from the communal area, examined, and administered treatment accordingly. Challenge tables should be cleaned and wiped down thoroughly between patients to limited risk for accidental exposure. The nurses station should be an area removed from patient access to reduce the risk of allergen cross-contamination and have space where food may be heated and measured. It also should be equipped with a small food scale, which may be necessary for graduated challenges, and be well stocked with clean, disposable plates, cups, and utensils.

AVOID DELAYS/FAILURES

Food allergies are associated with significant social and psychological consequences that often are overlooked by health care professionals. Anxiety and fear are so pervasive with this condition that many OFCs are cut short due to the inability of a patient or parent to proceed, often with no indication of a clinical reaction. Children and their parents report a range of psychosocial concerns that include parenting stress, fear of reaction, chronic anxiety around mealtime, depression, and worries about bullying. To avoid accidental exposures, some caregivers attempt to control their child's environment by limiting social interaction by home-schooling, forbidding sleepovers and birthday parties, avoiding traveling on airplanes, and not attending certain sporting events, all of which can be isolating for their food-allergic children. This hypervigilance can instill excessive amounts of anxiety and fear, which can affect all members of the family, food allergic or not.[37–39] For most families, the primary question that must be addressed is how to balance the vigilance and preparedness required of a potentially life-threatening chronic illness with anxiety management and engagement in developmentally appropriate activities.[40]

Addressing the psychological impact of food allergy for both patients and parents is an unmet need that needs to be addressed prior to any OFC in the office. Tackling these concerns early on will save valuable time in the future and help foster trust by normalizing parent and patient feelings. If symptoms are concerning enough, referral to a mental health professional for consultation is indicated to improve coping strategies and improve quality of life. Cognitive behavioral therapy is a well-validated, collaborative treatment that focuses on the relationships of thoughts, feelings, and behaviors. Cognitive behavioral therapy helps patients and parents identify patterns of thinking and behavior that contribute to distress and learn ways to change these patterns in a positive direction.[37,41]

To avoid OFC delays or failures related to increased anxiety and stress, an attempt must be made to create a relaxing, child-friendly environment. Tablets, toys, books, and other activities should be encouraged to aid in distracting patients during challenges and help avoid subjective complaints, which can often derail a challenge before it has the chance to get started. Parents should bring their child's favorite cups, plates, and utensils from home to create a sense of familiarity. There should be lots of food challenge options available in both liquid and solid forms along with tasty mixers and condiments to mask bad tastes, including ketchup, chocolate sauce, ice cream, applesauce, candy, and so forth. Infant challenges require additional preparation secondary to unique issues that arise due to their age and size (**Box 1**).[42]

PREPARE AND CONSENT

Preparing for a successful OFC in the office does not start the day of the challenge but instead starts at the initial consultation. Most of the time and effort should be spent at the initial visit beginning with a comprehensive medical history, including a detailed timeline of previous food reactions, amount of suspected food that was ingested, the form of food ingested (baked, raw, or canned), timing from ingestion to onset of symptoms, and whether the suspected food was tolerated without symptoms either before or since the reaction occurred. Reviewing changes of previous sIgE and/or skin tests over time provides more insight into disease progression and can help determine if a patient is a candidate for challenge. The final and most important

---

Box 1
Issues unique to infant oral food challenges

- Appropriate portion sizes for age
  - Portion size is more important than protein content.
  - Infant may not eat entire portion but may eat enough to rule out diagnosis.

- Appropriate vehicles/food forms
  - Soft/pureed
  - Avoid choking hazards (ie, peanut and tree nut kernels).
  - Have alternative food options available (ie, butters, puffs, and liquids).

- Provide mixing vehicles/condiments infant has previously tolerated.

- Allow ample time to feed.
  - Infants often dictate visit length so reserve plenty of time.

- Appropriate weight-based doses of emergency meds should be available.

- Familiarity with age-appropriate vital signs
  - Appropriately sized blood pressure cuffs

- OFC planned for a time of day when the infant is normally awake and alert
  - Avoid appointments during nap time.

Data from Greenhawt M. Pearls and pitfalls of food challenges in infants. Allergy Asthma Proc 2019;40(1):62-69.

step is educating the family on the nuances of a food allergy diagnosis, including everything from developing a food allergy and anaphylaxis emergency care plan, to how to read food labels, to ordering safe foods in restaurants and while traveling, to managing food allergy in school and daycare settings, and to knowing what cross-contamination exposures are worrisome and which are not. After determining that an in-office food challenge is indicated, specific questions should be addressed before the actual OFC appointment. Standard questions include:

1. What is an OFC?
2. What are the reasons to perform an OFC in the office versus at home?
3. What are the benefits?
4. What are the risks?
5. What needs to be done in preparation for an OFC?
   a. Medications that need to be stopped, including antihistamines
6. Who provides the food?
   a. Standardized recipes of baked milk and baked egg
   b. Bringing nut butters from sources where foods are not cross-contaminated
7. What happens the day of the challenge?
   a. Timing, sequence of events
   b. How long do I have to stay after challenge is completed?
   c. Make sure parents are aware of timeline; allocate approximately 4 hours to 6 hours.
8. What is the usual treatment in case of an allergic reaction?
9. If challenge is passed, how much and how often does food need to be ingested?

A phone call 1 day to 2 days prior to the OFC is important to confirm that the patient is well with no health issues that could affect interpretation of the challenge.[42] This is especially important in nonverbal infants where a concurrent illness during OFC could lower the threshold to react or increase the risk of a more severe reaction. Challenges should be scheduled in the morning or early afternoon so that patients have extra time in office for observation in case a reaction occurs. In preparation for the challenge, patients should not eat for at least 4 hours prior because fasting has been shown to enhance absorption of the challenged food.[36] For infants and toddlers, a light meal can be administered at approximately 2 hours before the challenge. It is important to time challenges to coincide with mealtimes, specifically breakfast or lunch. The concerning food served alongside chosen mixers or condiments can serve as a meal and improve chances of completing the challenge. Any food residue left on lips, face, and hands should be wiped off immediately to avoid contact irritation.

On the day of the challenge, baseline vital signs should be obtained, including respiratory rate, heart rate, blood pressure and peak flow if able. If the peak flow is low or there are concerns for asthma, a spirometry should be performed to exclude asthma. Patients with previously confirmed asthma should have a baseline spirometry prior to any challenges to confirm lung function is stable. Good asthma control prior to OFCs is essential for the safety of the patient. Optimizing control of other allergic conditions like allergic rhinitis and AD cannot be overlooked as well. Better control of atopy in general can minimize the risk of a severe reaction and limit variables that could affect interpretation of the challenge outcome. Physical examination findings should be documented as well to serve as a reference in case there are any changes during the challenge. Emergency medications should be readily accessible (high-risk challenges may have epinephrine drawn up and ready to go). Before proceeding, a standardized informed consent should be reviewed with the parents in detail and signed before any challenge takes place. It is the opinion of the author that written informed consent should be mandatory for any possible life-threatening procedure and should be standard practice in any office offering OFCs.

In addition to documentation of consent, OFC flow sheets/procedural forms should be meticulously maintained during the challenge. Detailed recordings of time, doses, vital signs, symptoms, and intervening treatments improve safety and accuracy of the challenge and provide a historical record that can be referred to in the future if needed. Timers can be used to keep challenges on track, especially in busy practices where multiple food challenges are taking place at the same time.

PREASSIGNED ROLES

To streamline efficiency and improve safety of OFCs, there needs to be clear, defined roles for the entire treatment team. In busy offices, preassigned roles limit errors and

---

Box 2
Proposed stopping criteria infant peanut oral food challenge for early peanut introduction

Adverse Reactions to Foods Committee of the AAAAI proposed food challenge stopping criteria[a]

The OFC should be stopped if any one of the following symptoms are present during the OFC:
Skin
- ≥3 urticarial lesions
- Angioedema
- Confluent erythematous, pruritic rash

Respiratory
- Wheezing
- Repetitive cough
- Difficulty breathing/increased work of breathing
- Stridor
- Dysphonia
- Aphonia

Gastrointestinal
- Vomiting alone not associated with gag reflex
- Severe abdominal pain (such as abnormal stillness, inconsolable crying, or drawing legs up to abdomen) that persists for ≥3 minutes

Cardiovascular
- Hypotension for age not associated with vasovagal episode

If 2 or more of the following are present, the OFC should be stopped:
Skin
- Persistent scratching for ≥3 minutes

Respiratory
- Persistent rubbing of the nose or eye for ≥3 minutes
- Persistent rhinorrhea for ≥3 minutes

Gastrointestinal
- Diarrhea

Can be generalized to any infant challenge.
Suggested food challenge stopping criteria from the Adverse Reactions to Foods Committee of the AAAAI.

[a] It is important to note that the physician is encouraged to use discretion and clinical judgment when assessing the challenge outcome. Whenever observed signs or symptoms are inconclusive. it may be appropriate for the clinician performing the challenge to decide if a challenge dose should be repeated, the next dose should be delayed, or if the challenge should be stopped and repeated on another day. If clinically indicated, dosing is stopped. Objective symptoms that recur on 3 doses or persist (eg, 40 minutes) are more likely indicative of a reaction than when such symptoms are transient and not reproducible.

From Bird JA, Groetch M, Allen KJ, et al. Conducting an Oral Food Challenge to Peanut in an Infant. J Allergy Clin Immunol Pract 2017;5(2):309; with permission.

allow clinics to accommodate multiple food challenges at once. Specific roles can include determining who prepares and divides up the food for challenge, who performs vital signs and assesses symptoms, who administers doses, and who administers treatments should a reaction occur. The patient should be closely monitored throughout the duration of OFC, with re-examination at regular intervals by experienced observers trained in OFCs. At the first sign/symptom of an allergic reaction, a physical examination should be performed and include auscultation of the chest, inspection of the skin and oropharynx, and repeat vital signs and peak flow. Subjective complaints are common, especially with the first few doses. Classic symptoms include nausea and throat, mouth, and skin itch as well as a sensation of throat tightness or globus sensation (usually with no other findings). For mild symptoms, a period of observation should be allowed before giving the next dose. Administering epinephrine at the first sign of a reaction should be avoided if criteria have not been met for anaphylaxis. There also should be clearly determined stopping criteria and a standardized treatment approach for all patients, with a plan on how to transfer patients to the emergency room in refractory cases (**Box 2**).[43] In group practices, assessing providers should agree with these criteria to avoid confusion among ancillary staff. OFCs are not always clear-cut, so questionable reactions can be treated at the discretion of the physician. The supervising physician should always be onsite for OFCs and perform the prechallenge examination as well as be available for any reactions should they occur. In a busy practice, limiting disruptions to patient flow is important, but staff should feel free to interrupt the treating physician if any concerns arise during a challenge. Every effort should be made to standardize and streamline OFC procedures to limit confusion, provide continuity among providers, and maximize safety. Standardized approaches should be used when administering food using premeasured doses as well as standardized protocols for stopping and treating any reactions should they occur. Clear, well-understood, prespecified stopping criteria is a key safety feature in published clinical trials and likely contributed to the low rates of anaphylaxis reported.

If the OFC is successful, clear postchallenge instructions should be provided to the parents encouraging regular consumption at home. This is especially true if baked challenges are completed, so parents know what foods are safe and what foods still need to be avoided. There are few data regarding the appropriate amount of the allergenic food that needs to be ingested after a successful OFC. Based on available evidence and consensus opinion, regular consumption at least 3 days a week is recommended.[43] In rare situations, there can be relapse in children who pass a challenge but fail to consistently incorporate concerning foods into their diet, so follow-up in 3 months to 6 months is recommended to reinforce the importance of regular ingestion.[16,43,44]

FUTURE CONSIDERATIONS

Although the need for OFCs continues to increase, there seems to be an increasing reluctance to offer them in clinical practices. This trend was demonstrated in a workgroup report from the American Academy of Allergy, Asthma & Immunology (AAAAI) Adverse Reactions to Foods Committee (ARFC).[45] A survey was provided to both AAAAI and American College of Allergy, Asthma & Immunology (ACAAI) members looking at OFC practices among allergists in the United States. It was based on a food allergy survey administered by Pongracic and colleagues in 2009 that was updated to reflect recent advances in food allergy and knowledge gaps that were not addressed in previous survey, such as OFCs in very young children.[46] Compared to 2009, while more providers offer OFCs, multiple perceived barriers to performing OFCs have worsened over time including lack of time, experience, staff, and office space. These concerns were heightened in the infant patient population with an emerging pattern of hesitancy to challenge infants despite nearly all respondents reporting seeing patients <12 months of age in their practice. The demand for OFCs in infants and toddlers will likely continue to increase, and existing guidelines (as defined in the National Institutes of Allergy and Infectious Diseases addendum guidelines) are predicated on both access and willingness to perform OFCs in this age group. Additional follow-up surveys related to hesitancy for performing infant OFCs will likely be pursued in order to further clarify barriers and other safety concerns in this age group.

SUMMARY

Food challenges in infants and toddlers seem to be safe when looking at the available data for both high-risk patients with prior history of reactions and infants with no known exposure to the food being challenged. The benefits of OFCs are far reaching and impactful for both patients and their parents. Improvement in quality of life, clarifying unnecessary dietary restrictions, increased social interactions, and reduction in fear and anxiety are just a few of the many advantages of providing this service. Demand for OFCs in infants and toddlers will continue to increase in the coming years. Board-certified allergists will need to meet these demands by providing this service in a safe and welcoming environment. The barriers discussed in the recent ARFC survey need to be addressed, including more comprehensive food challenge education and hands-on experience during fellowship training, so patients can receive the care they deserve.

REFERENCES

1. Simons FE, Sampson HA. Anaphylaxis: Unique aspects of clinical diagnosis and management in infants (birth to age 2 years). J Allergy Clin Immunol 2015;135: 1125–31.
2. Palmer DJ, Sullivan TR, Gold MS, et al. Randomized controlled trial of early regular egg intake to prevent egg allergy. J Allergy Clin Immunol 2017;139: 1600–7.e2.
3. Wei-Liang Tan J, Valerio C, Barnes EH, et al. A randomized trial of egg introduction from 4 months of age in infants at risk for egg allergy. J Allergy Clin Immunol 2017;139:1621–8.e8.
4. Bellach J, Schwarz V, Ahrens B, et al. Randomized placebo-controlled trial of hen's egg consumption for primary prevention in infants. J Allergy Clin Immunol 2017;139:1591–9.e2.
5. Mankad VS, Williams LW, Lee LA, et al. Safety of open food challenges in the office setting. Ann Allergy Asthma Immunol 2008;100:469–74.
6. Akuete K, Guffey D, Israelsen RB, et al. Multicenter prevalence of anaphylaxis in clinic-based oral food challenges. Ann Allergy Asthma Immunol 2017;119(4): 339–48.e1.
7. Fleischer DM, Bock SA, Spears GC, et al. Oral food challenges in children with a diagnosis of food allergy. J Pediatr 2011;158:578–83.
8. Noone S, Ross J, Sampson HA, et al. Epinephrine use in positive oral food challenges performed as a screening test for food allergy therapy trials. J Allergy Clin Immunol Pract 2015;3:424–8.
9. Lieberman JA, Cox AL, Vitale M, et al. Outcomes of office-based, open food challenges in the management of food allergy. J Allergy Clin Immunol 2011;128: 1120–2.

10. Perry TT, Matsui EC, Conover-Walker MK, et al. Risk of oral food challenges. J Allergy Clin Immunol 2004;114:1164–8.

11. Ram G, Cianferoni A, Spergel JM. Food allergy to uncommonly challenged foods is rare based on oral food challenge. J Allergy Clin Immunol Pract 2016;4: 156–7.e5.

12. Järvinen KM, Amalanayagam S, Shreffler WG, et al. Epinephrine treatment is infrequent and biphasic reactions are rare in food-induced reactions during oral food challenges in children. J Allergy Clin Immunol 2009;124:1267–72.

13. Lee J, Garrett JP, Brown-Whitehorn T, et al. Biphasic reactions in children undergoing oral food challenges. Allergy Asthma Proc 2013;34:220–6.

14. Osborne NJ, Koplin JJ, Martin PE, et al. Prevalence of challenge-proven IgE-mediated food allergy using population-based sampling and predetermined challenge criteria in infants. J Allergy Clin Immunol 2011;127:668–76.e1-2.

15. Clopton, J. (2017, August 8). Alabama Boy's Death Worries Food Allergy Parents. WebMD Health News. Retrieved from https://www.webmd.com/allergies/news/20170807/alabama-boys-death-worries-food-allergy-parents.

16. Du Toit G, Roberts G, Sayre PH, et al. Randomized trial of peanut consumption in infants at risk for peanut allergy. N Engl J Med 2015;372:803–13.

17. Perkin MR, Logan K, Tseng A, et al. Randomized trial of introduction of allergenic foods in breast-fed infants. N Engl J Med 2016;374:1733–43.

18. Perry TT, Matsui EC, Kay Conover-Walker M, et al. The relationship of allergen-specific IgE levels and oral food challenge outcome. J Allergy Clin Immunol 2004;114:144–9.

19. Sampson HA. Food allergy. Part 2: diagnosis and management. J Allergy Clin Immunol 1999;103:981–99.

20. Shek LPC, Soderstrom L, Ahlstedt S, et al. Determination of food specific IgE levels over time can predict the development of tolerance in cow's milk and hen's egg allergy. J Allergy Clin Immunol 2004;114:387–91.

21. Ho MH, Wong WH, Heine RG, et al. Early clinical predictors of remission of peanut allergy in children. J Allergy Clin Immunol 2008;121:731–6.

22. Savage J, Sicherer S, Wood R. The natural history of food allergy. J Allergy Clin Immunol Pract 2016;4:196–203.

23. Santos AF, Brough HA. Making the most of in vitro tests to diagnose food allergy. J Allergy Clin Immunol Pract 2017;5(2):237–48.

24. Simberloff T, Parambi R, Bartnikas LM, et al. Implementation of a standardized clinical assessment and management plan (SCAMP) for food challenges. J Allergy Clin Immunol Pract 2017;5(2):335–44.

25. Frischmeyer-Guerrerio PA, Rasooly M, Gu W, et al. IgE testing can predict food allergy status in patients with moderate to severe atopic dermatitis. Ann Allergy Asthma Immunol 2019;122(4):393–400.

26. Urisu A, Yamada K, Tokuda R, et al. Clinical significance of IgE-binding activity to enzymatic digests of ovomucoid in the diagnosis and the prediction of the outgrowing of egg white hypersensitivity. Int Arch Allergy Immunol 1999;120: 192–8.

27. Nicolaou N, Murray C, Belgrave D, et al. Quantification of specific IgE to whole peanut extract and peanut components in prediction of peanut allergy. J Allergy Clin Immunol 2011;127:684–5.

28. Tuano KS, Davis CM. Utility of component-resolved diagnostics in food allergy. Curr Allergy Asthma Rep 2015;15:32.

29. Caubet JC, Bencharitiwong R, Moshier E, et al. Significance of ovomucoid- and ovalbumin-specific IgE/IgG(4) ratios in egg allergy. J Allergy Clin Immunol 2012; 129:739–47.
30. Santos AF, Douiri A, Becares N, et al. Basophil activation test discriminates between allergy and tolerance in peanut sensitized children. J Allergy Clin Immunol 2014;134:645–52.
31. Santos AF, Du Toit G, Douiri A, et al. Distinct parameters of the basophil activation test reflect the severity and threshold of allergic reactions to peanut. J Allergy Clin Immunol 2015;135:179–86.
32. Konstantinou GN, Nowak-Wegrzyn A, Bencharitiwong R, et al. Egg-white-specific IgA and IgA2 antibodies in egg allergic children: is there a role in tolerance induction? Pediatr Allergy Immunol 2014;25:64–70.
33. Rolinck-Werninghaus C, Niggemann B, Grabenhenrich L, et al. Outcome of oral food challenges in children in relation to symptom-eliciting allergen dose and allergen-specific IgE. Allergy 2012;67:951–7.
34. DunnGalvin A, Daly D, Cullinane C, et al. Highly accurate prediction of food challenge outcome using routinely available clinical data. J Allergy Clin Immunol 2011;127:633–9.e1-3.
35. Sampson HA, Ho DG. Relationship between food-specfic IgE concentrations and the risk of positive food challenges in children and adolescents. J Allergy Clin Immunol 1997;100:444–51.
36. Nowak-Wegrzyn A, Assa'ad AH, Bahna SL, et al. Work Group report: oral food challenge testing. J Allergy Clin Immunol 2009;123:S365–83.
37. Cummings AJ, Knibb RC, King RM, et al. The psychosocial impact of food allergy and food hypersensitivity in children, adolescents, and their families: a review. Allergy 2010;65:933–45.
38. Ravid NL, Annunziato RA, Ambrose MA, et al. Mental health and quality-of-life concerns related to the burden of food allergy. Immunol Allergy Clin North Am 2012;32:83–95.
39. Lieberman JA, Sicherer SH. Quality of life in food allergy. Curr Opin Allergy Clin Immunol 2011;11:236–42.
40. Herbert L, Shemesh E, Bender B. Clinical management of psychosocial concerns related to food allergy. J Allergy Clin Immunol Pract 2016;4(2):205–13.
41. Knibb RC. Effectiveness of cognitive behaviour therapy for mothers of children with food allergy: a case series. Healthcare (Basel) 2015;3(4):1194–211.
42. Greenhawt M. Pearls and pitfalls of food challenges in infants. Allergy Asthma Proc 2019;40(1):62–9.
43. Bird JA, Groetch M, Allen KJ, et al. Conducting an oral food challenge to peanut in an infant. J Allergy Clin Immunol Pract 2017;5(2):301–11.
44. Fleischer DM, Conover-Walker MK, Christie L, et al. The natural progression of peanut allergy: resolution and the possibility of recurrence. J Allergy Clin Immunol 2003;112:183–9.
45. Greiwe J, Oppenheimer J, Fleischer DM, et al. AAAAI AFRC workgroup report: oral food challenge practices among allergists in the United States. Manuscript in preparation.
46. Pongracic JA, Bock SA, Sicherer SH. Oral food challenge practices among allergists in the United States. J Allergy Clin Immunol 2012;129:564–6.

Moving Past "Avoid All Nuts"

Individualizing Management of Children with Peanut/Tree Nut Allergies

Brian Schroer, MD[a],*, Jaclyn Bjelac, MD[b]

KEYWORDS

- Peanut allergy • Tree nuts • Unnecessary avoidance • Food allergy prevention
- Collaborative decision making

KEY POINTS

- Avoiding tree nuts in patients with peanut allergy is a choice that needs to be made by the family after being counseled about the benefits and risks of the potential decisions.
- In patients who are at high risk for developing food allergies, unnecessary food avoidance may increase the risk for patients to become allergic to that food.
- Families should decide whether they desire screening for food sensitization before ingestion of the food.
- The main goal for allergists and families should be to prevent food allergies.
- Prevention of food allergies requires a collaborative approach to safely allow families to introduce allergenic foods in children who are at high risk.

CASE PRESENTATION

Emily is a 9-month-old patient who presents to the clinic for evaluation of possible peanut allergy. She has a history of early-onset moderate eczema, which has been well controlled with skin hygiene measures and twice-weekly application of prescription strength topical steroid ointment. Two weeks before the allergy visit she ate peanut for the first time. She ingested 2 bites of peanut butter mixed with applesauce and developed almost immediate hives on her face, chin, and neck. She was then noted to sneeze. Her mother wiped off her face and gave her diphenhydramine. Her mother reports that 15 minutes after ingestion, Emily had a single episode of emesis. No further symptoms developed, and hives and sneezing resolved within 45 minutes of onset. They have since continued to avoid peanuts. When they come to the office, her

Disclosure: The authors have nothing to disclose.
[a] Akron Children's Hospital, 130 West Exchange Street, Akron, OH 44022, USA; [b] Cleveland Clinic Children's Hospital, 9500 Euclid Avenue, A3, Cleveland, OH 44195, USA
* Corresponding author.
E-mail address: bschroer@akronchildrens.org

Immunol Allergy Clin N Am 39 (2019) 495–506
https://doi.org/10.1016/j.iac.2019.07.004
0889-8561/19/© 2019 Elsevier Inc. All rights reserved.

parents report that Emily has never ingested a tree nut. They have read on social media that many parents are introducing tree nuts to their children with eczema or other food allergies, stating that doing so would prevent tree nut allergy. Before testing for peanut, the doctor had a conversation with the family that included a discussion of whether or not patients with peanut allergy have to avoid all nuts, and what testing may be appropriate during this visit.

This article covers the evidence for why recommendations to avoid all nuts in someone with a single nut allergy are changing, and reviews options for select nut introduction in children with peanut or tree nut allergy.

AVOIDING ALL NUTS IF ALLERGIC TO 1

Peanut and tree nut allergies are among the most common causes of food allergy in the United States,[1] and food allergy significantly affects quality of life for children and their families.[2] Historically, it was common for a child with 1 food allergy to undergo additional testing to other common food allergens, even without a history of reaction. The justification was presumably to prevent the children from having a reaction to other foods the first time they were consumed in an unsupervised setting. Although this approach was intended for patient protection, there was a high potential for unnecessary avoidance of food given the possibility of false-positive testing.[3] In patients with peanut allergy, tree nut allergy testing before introduction has been common. Expert opinion has been to have all peanut-allergic patients avoid tree nuts despite the lack of a history of a reaction to tree nuts.[4] This recommendation was based on anecdotal reports of peanut-allergic children reacting to tree nuts because of cross-contact with peanut.[5]

PEANUTS VERSUS TREE NUTS

Peanuts are a legume. Although their name contains the word nut, they differ botanically from tree nuts such as cashew, pistachio, walnut, pecan, almond, hazelnut, and Brazil nuts. Despite differing taxonomy, previously published reports suggest a 30% chance of cosensitization and potential for a reaction to tree nuts in peanut-allergic children.[5] With this information, historically many patients with peanut allergy were advised to avoid tree nuts. This form of patient protection has typically been done without a conversation with the family about whether it was an option to learn how to identify tree nuts, read labels, and search for manufacturers of tree nuts that do not have potential cross-contact with peanut.

Recent articles suggest that the rates of coallergy to tree nuts in peanut-allergic patients may be lower than previously reported.[6] The HealthNuts prospective study from Australia shows that children who had peanut allergy at 1 year old had a 27% chance of having challenge-confirmed tree nut allergy at 6 years old.[7] So far, the evidence for avoiding all tree nuts in someone diagnosed with peanut anaphylaxis has been based on expert opinion with little evidence to support a single correct approach.[8] It should also be noted that, in peanut-allergic or tree nut–allergic children, introduction of specific nuts to which the child is not allergic may improve quality of life and allow dietary expansion.[9]

WHY NOT AVOID ALL NUTS IF ALLERGIC TO 1?

At the moment, the practice of avoiding all nuts if allergic to 1 is changing for many reasons. Some of the impetus for changing this practice is the recognition that both skin prick testing (SPT) and serum specific IgE (sIgE) testing lead to many false-positives.[10] These tests have a high negative predictive value and a poor positive predictive value. In all patients, a history of any prior reaction or tolerance of ingestion of a typical serving remains the ultimate test. Using tests alone to diagnose tree nut allergy increases the risk that patients are avoiding these tree nuts unnecessarily.

RISK OF UNNECESSARY AVOIDANCE?

In 2015, the Learning Early About Peanut (LEAP) trial changed management of food allergy by showing that early introduction of peanut and ingesting it 3 times per week significantly decreases the risk of becoming allergic in children deemed to be at high risk of developing peanut allergy.[11] All patients in the trial were at high risk for food allergies because of having either moderate to severe eczema or egg allergy. One group of children who had negative allergy skin prick tests to peanut ate peanut early, leading to an 86.1% relative risk reduction for becoming allergic. The other group of children LEAP studied had positive skin or blood testing but passed a peanut ingestion challenge. In this group, eating peanut early and often led to a relative risk reduction for developing a peanut allergy of 70.0%.[11] Although there is only 1 study showing this benefit in peanut, studies have shown that early introduction of egg in high-risk individuals can decrease the risk of developing egg allergy.[12] Looking at these studies a different way, this same evidence suggests that unnecessarily avoiding allergenic foods such as peanut or egg in children who are not clinically allergic may contribute to developing allergies to those foods.

EATING ALLERGENIC FOODS TO PREVENT FOOD ALLERGY

The evolving knowledge that unnecessary food avoidance may be a factor contributing to development of food allergy has led many allergists to realize that their goal should be to facilitate introduction of allergenic foods into the diets of children who are at high risk for becoming allergic. There are data to support early introduction of selected allergenic foods in the diet that show both efficacy for egg and peanut introduction and a lack of harm with this approach for milk, wheat, sesame, and whitefish in a normal-risk population.[13,14] However, such data are lacking for tree nuts.[8] Prevention of tree nut allergy would be an important goal because most patients who develop a tree nut allergy never outgrow it.[15] In the absence of specific evidence showing benefit or risk for early introduction of foods beyond egg and peanut, it is necessary for allergists to have a relationship-centered discussion with families of patients with food allergy about how to safely introduce other allergenic foods.[16]

HOW TO INTRODUCE ALLERGENIC FOODS IN HIGH-RISK CHILDREN

Publication of the LEAP study results, multiple society guidelines have been published regarding how to implement early peanut introduction. However, there are many questions about how to implement this evidence at a population level. One controversy centers on the necessity of prescreening before introduction of peanut. Recommendations differ between guidelines. In the United States, the National Institute of Allergy and Infectious Diseases (NIAID)/National Institutes of Health recommend prescreening using either SPT or sIgE testing before peanut introduction in select children.[17] The recommendations from the British Society of Allergy and Clinical Immunology (BSACI) do not recommend routine prescreening when introducing peanut, even in high-risk children.[18] The Australian Society of Clinical Immunology and Allergy (ASCIA) guidelines written in 2016 state that introduction of foods such as egg, peanut, and tree nuts should not be delayed and do not mention prescreening even a high-risk population, suggesting those patients at high risk discuss their preferred approach with their doctors.[19]

TESTING BEFORE INGESTION

The most notable potential benefit in recommending preintroduction screening evaluation is minimizing the number of children who react to peanut in an unsupervised setting at the time of first introduction at home. However, there are known and potential risks of routinely recommending prescreening before introduction of peanut or other allergenic foods, even in high-risk populations. The known risk is the cost of screening.[20] A study from Australia on the feasibility of implementing LEAP-style peanut introduction in the high-risk group estimated that 16% of the population would require screening before peanut ingestion.[21] Of these high-risk patients, their data show that 13.4% would require an in-office challenge if all with SPT wheals of 3 to 7 mm were challenged. Another risk is that prescreening in selected populations may still miss patients who are already allergic. The same study showed that screening these patients would still miss an estimated 23% of children with peanut allergy in the lower risk group.[21] Their data also suggest that introduction of peanut without prescreening in the high-risk group is safe because, in the 185 high-risk infants who introduced peanut on their own (a self-selected population) before 12 months of age, only 1 had symptoms consistent with possible anaphylaxis. That patient is reported to have passed an in-office challenge 2 months later.[21]

An unknown risk is that children who would have introduced peanut into their diets before publication of such guidelines are deterred from doing so by a lack of resources or experts who are able to adequately implement prescreening recommendations.[20] In addition, it is not clear how many patients who are screened and found to have positive skin or blood testing are offered and then actually undergo food challenges, even if the results indicate a low risk of clinical allergy.[20] The investigators suggest that prescreening potentially, "results in a paradoxical effect, where over proscriptive [sic] guidelines to support early introduction have the opposite effect and increase the risk of food allergy in later life."[20] The cost-effectiveness, benefits, and risks of routine prescreening before introduction of foods such as peanut require extensive prospective studies to answer many remaining questions. These studies would be necessary for tree nuts as well.

CASE EXAMPLE

Applying this concept to Emily, it is possible that prescreening for tree nut could paradoxically lead to tree nut allergy. Suppose that her family had been planning to give Emily safe forms of tree nuts and she is not clinically allergic. However, because of her peanut allergy, she is screened and found to be positive to walnut/pecan and cashew/pistachio at low levels. As a result of this testing they are told to avoid the walnuts/pecans, and cashews/pistachios until a physician-supervised in-office challenge can be accomplished. Because of a multitude of factors, including time constraints, fear, and costs related to the visit, they do not schedule a challenge. At follow-up 4 years later, they describe a recent reaction to walnuts involving full-body hives and vomiting after eating a few bites of a walnut-containing brownie. In this scenario, it could be argued that the screening may have contributed to the development of tree nut allergy because nut avoidance prevented the development of tolerance. The potential for risk of developing an allergy when avoiding tree nuts in patients who are sensitized without clinical allergy is not known.

DISCUSSION WITH FAMILIES ABOUT TESTING BEFORE INTRODUCTION

Although the guidelines noted earlier can be useful to assist in deciding whether to perform preintroduction screening for peanut, there are currently no published guidelines addressing this question for other commonly allergenic foods. The investigators of LEAP and other leaders in food allergy research discuss that there remains significant debate about the risks and benefits for screening before ingestion of peanut.[22] Because of this uncertainty, any decision to test for foods other than peanut in high-risk children is not supported by any evidence or clinical guidelines. Therefore, the decision about prescreening for tree nuts should be made as a joint decision of the family and the clinician.

CASE UPDATE

Before testing to peanut, Emily's family was given a few choices about whether to test for tree nuts simultaneously. This discussion included characterizing the skin tests as being very good at showing that she is not allergic if the tests for tree nuts are negative, but that a positive test does not necessarily means she is allergic. They are informed that any positive skin testing would be followed by in vitro testing, and potentially may lead to a several-hour in-office food challenge. Using a collaborative dialogue, they are given options for introduction of tree nuts in the peanut-allergic child at home.[16]

Emily's parents question the potential for a reaction to tree nut should they try them at home. They are told that up to 30% of peanut-allergic patients develop a tree nut allergy by 6 year old, and that although 31% of peanut-allergic children are sensitized to tree nuts at 1 year of age, it is unclear how many of these children are allergic.[7] It is important to also discuss the potential that unnecessary avoidance of tree nut has the potential to increase the risk of allergy.[23] Emily's parents are asked about their comfort with introducing tree nuts at home without testing, because it has been shown that anxiety modulates food selection in peanut-allergic patients. This conversation will clarify the family's perspective and facilitate an agreed-on plan of action.[24]

Based on this discussion, the family is asked to choose from a few options (**Fig. 1**):

1. Introduce tree nuts without prescreening before introduction
2. Perform prescreening with SPT or in vitro sIgE testing for tree nuts before introduction
3. Avoid all tree nuts in addition to peanut regardless of testing

IMPLEMENTING WHAT THE FAMILY WANTS

After discussion, many families elect to pursue introduction of tree nuts without screening for sensitization. This option may be selected by families who wish to liberalize their children's diets to include a variety of peanut alternatives, and who wish to avoid testing. It is important to assess the family's commitment to doing the introduction.

An alternative approach is to introduce tree nuts to the peanut-allergic child, with preintroduction testing. More risk-averse families may choose testing as a means to risk stratify further before introduction. Families should be permitted to make a decision regarding such testing following a discussion of the characteristics of currently available methods. This discussion should emphasize the low false-negative rates but also high rates of false-positives seen with both percutaneous and in vitro methods.[10] Specifically, peanut allergens do have some cross reactivity with tree nut allergens and therefore the tree nut allergy tests can be positive because of the peanut allergy but do not necessarily mean the child is allergic.[25] Before testing is accomplished, it is

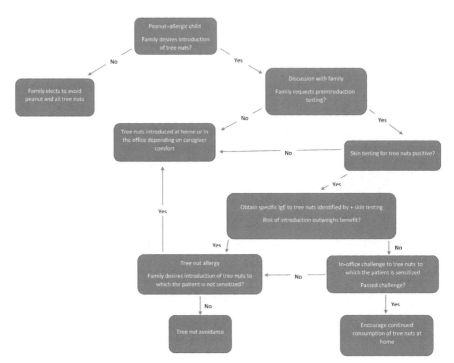

Fig. 1. Decision tree for deciding how to introduce tree nuts in a food-allergic child.

necessary to discuss with the families what will be recommended should the results be negative or positive. They should be counseled that negative testing indicates a low but not zero risk of reaction, and that a positive test would require additional evaluation and introduction of the food during an in-office oral food challenge. Clinicians should also discuss that risk stratification for positive testing is complicated by lack of population-based cutoffs for skin or serum testing to tree nuts.[6]

Avoidance of all tree nuts in addition to peanut is an option selected by some families. Families may choose this path for a variety of reasons, and understanding their perspective is important to implementing their preferences. Some families have concerns regarding peanut cross-contact with a given tree nut, and want to avoid all nuts because of the potential increased risk of accidental exposure to peanut. Although the published rate of peanut contamination in snack foods with precautionary allergy labeling ranges from 0.9% to 32.4%, peanut contamination in nonsnack items is far less common.[9] Particularly in very young children, families may wish to pursue this approach until the child is old enough to verbalize reaction symptoms or be able to question food contents. Prescreening for sensitivity would not be required at this time but could be considered in the future should the family pursue tree nut introduction.

Regardless of their decision, every effort should be made to assist the family in choosing a path with which they are comfortable, because reservations are likely to result in failure to introduce the food at home.

AFTER TESTING TO TREE NUTS

Should skin testing be pursued and sensitivity to 1 or more tree nuts be identified, a physician-supervised in-office challenge should be pursued. If desired, serum sIgE allows further risk stratification before the in-office challenge. Because cutoff values for tree nuts are not as well established as for peanut, and without a history of a reaction, an in-office physician-supervised food challenge should be offered to the tree nuts in question unless a high level of sensitivity suggests the risk would outweigh the benefit. The decision to undergo the challenge should be made in a collaborative fashion, discussing the benefits and potential risks. In patients with multiple positives to tree nuts, the possibility of multiple in-office challenges can be a barrier for patients and families. Cross reactivity has been identified among the tree nuts,[9,25,26] and this can be used to perform challenges to 2 or more tree nuts on a given challenge day.[27]

If allergy is diagnosed to 1 or more tree nuts, again the family is faced with the decision of whether to avoid all tree nuts, or just the tree nuts to which the child is allergic. The family should be encouraged to allow their child to consume tree nuts to which they are not allergic if desired, following counseling on the necessity of obtaining tree nuts not contaminated with the known allergen.

If testing is done and is negative, the family should be asked to relay the results of the at-home challenge. If any reactions occur, they should return for a follow-up for evaluation and management for this tree nut allergy.

CASE UPDATE: EMILY'S FAMILY DECISION

When presented with these 3 options, Emily's parents decide to pursue testing only to peanut. They are comfortable that they can recognize and treat a reaction because they have self-injectable epinephrine and they were told they will receive further education on how to recognize and treat a reaction at the end of the visit. Skin testing to peanut was positive at 6×27-mm wheal/flare and her sIgE to peanut is 5.67 kU/L with Ara h 2 of 4.54 kU/L. Based on her reaction and confirmatory testing, Emily is diagnosed with peanut allergy. The family is educated on avoidance measures, and a food allergy action plan is reviewed. When being instructed on how to introduce tree nuts, they are told to do an at-home graded introduction of a tree nut. Once the nuts have been introduced without reaction, they are instructed to have Emily ingest them regularly, at least weekly, even though the allergist admits there is no published guidance on how often the tree nuts need to be eaten for tolerance to be maintained.

AFTER THE VISIT: INTRODUCTION AT HOME

When testing is not pursued, guidance should be provided to families on how to safely introduce the tree nuts at home. There is no clear guidance on how to do this. It is reasonable to suggest an at-home graded-dose challenge similar to the recommendations for at-home peanut introduction. Patients can use finely chopped or butter forms of tree nuts that can be mixed with age-appropriate foods such as fruit purees. A small amount can be eaten and then monitored for a set period of time. When no reaction occurs, the clinician can recommend various options, including slow introduction of a serving or a multiple-step graded-dose challenge based on the family's preferences. The family should be told to do this introduction on a day when they are not distracted so that they can recognize and treat any reactions. By having a dialogue about how to introduce tree nuts at home, patients can ask questions and the clinician can identify and address any barriers to tree nut introduction.

ADDRESSING QUESTIONS AND CONCERNS

At the end of a clinic visit, the family's ability and comfort with implementing these options should be assessed using open-ended questions. If people initially indicated they did not want testing but then say that they are not likely to introduce any tree nuts at home without risk stratification, then testing should be discussed again. Other common questions or concerns that arise include, but are not limited to: how to find tree nuts that are not contaminated by peanut, whether any peanut residue can be washed off tree nuts, how to recognize various tree nuts, what to tell schools or restaurants, how to give children these tree nuts regularly, whether any future siblings need to be tested before peanut or tree nut introduction, what to do if another sibling in the family has a tree nut allergy, and what needs to be done for an older child with peanut allergy who has always avoided tree nuts. A theme of this topic is that there remains little evidence and few guidelines about how to answer these questions.

PEANUT CROSS-CONTACT IN TREE NUTS

When it comes to finding tree nuts that do not contain any peanut protein or residue from cross contact, parents should be advised that all individually packed forms of tree nuts need to be assessed on a case-by-case basis. As is the case with most food allergies, it is imperative for families and patients to be able to read labels and understand the need to avoid products that use precautionary labels. The need to avoid precautionary labels may significantly limit the ability of families to find forms of peanut-free tree nuts. That situation has led some people to inquire about the effect of buying potentially contaminated nuts and washing any peanut residue off. Although it is possible that water rinses may remove peanut allergen, no study has been done to prove that this is a safe option.

MIXED-UP NUTS

There is evidence that both allergists and patients with food allergies have trouble visually identifying different tree nuts. Patients should be told that learning how to recognize different tree nuts is beneficial when eating some tree nuts but avoiding others[28] (**Fig. 2**, **Table 1**). All caregivers for these children should be educated about how to avoid the allergenic foods and how to safely serve the tolerated tree nuts. They should be counseled that many restaurant and food service workers have little training in food allergen identification and avoidance strategies.[29] Asking schools or teachers

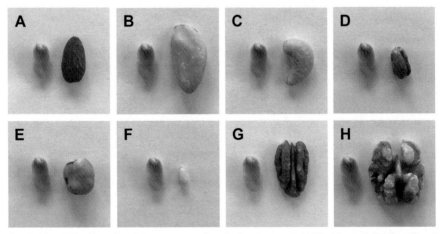

Fig. 2. Identification of various tree nuts in relation to peanut. (*A*) Almond. (*B*) Brazil nut. (*C*) Cashew. (*D*) Pistachio. (*E*) Filbert. (*F*) Pine nut. (*G*) Pecan. (*H*) Walnut.

Table 1	
Nut allergy co-occurrence	
Primary Nut Allergen	**Most Common Co-occurring Nut Allergens**
Pecan[a]	Walnut,[a] peanut
Pistachio[a]	Cashew[a]
Hazelnut	Macadamia nut
Brazil nut	Macadamia nut

[a] In the referenced study, 16.7% of cashew-allergic children were not allergic to pistachio, although only 2.8% of children allergic to pistachio were not allergic to cashew. Nearly 30% of children allergic to walnut were not allergic to pecan, although just 6.1% of pecan-allergic patients were not allergic to walnut.

Data from Brough HA, Caubet J, Mazon A, et al. Abstract 0124: Peanut, tree-nut and sesame seedallergies: do children allergic to a nut or sesameseed need to avoid all nuts? Special Issue: Abstracts from the European Academy of Allergy and Clinical Immunology Congress, 17–21 June 2017, Helsinki, Finland. Allergy European Journal of Allergy and Clinical Immunology; Volume 72, Issue S103: pages 103-104.

to understand that a child has to avoid peanut but can eat tree nuts requires individual and specific discussions and should be done on a case-by-case basis. Because of these issues, it may be best if patients limit the ingestion of nonallergenic nuts to the home, where trusted caregivers know what foods to avoid and what is safe to ingest.

HOW OFTEN DO THEY NEED TO EAT TREE NUTS?

Whether all of these tree nuts need to be ingested regularly, and, if so, how often, remains a question. It may be assumed that patients should be told to ingest tree nuts 3 times per week, similar to what is recommended by the NIAID for peanuts. If this is the case, then eating almonds, hazelnuts, cashews, pistachios, pecans, walnuts, and peanuts multiple times weekly may be difficult to implement on a routine basis. In the United States, walnut, pecan, cashews, and pistachios cause the most tree nut allergies.[30] Focusing regular ingestion on the most common tree nuts to cause allergy may facilitate regular ingestion of those nuts. One option that can make it easier to give multiple nuts at 1 time is using multinut butters. By using a multinut butter, 1 serving covers all of the nuts that need to be eaten regularly. To decrease expense, patients are sharing recipes for home production of multinut butters on food allergy support groups on social media. Commercially prepared multinut butters are also available.

TESTING SIBLINGS

When prescreening children whose siblings are known to be peanut allergic, families should be counseled that the current NIAID practice parameter does not recommend prescreening testing in siblings of patients with peanut allergy. It is necessary to understand the family's perspective, assess for any questions or barriers to feeling comfortable to introduce without testing, and then provide specific information to address these concerns. If the family continues to have reservations about introduction without such testing, then testing before introduction should be offered.

TREE NUTS IN THE HOUSE WHEN OTHER PEOPLE ARE ALLERGIC

Another concern expressed by many families is reservations about the presence of peanut or tree nuts in the home as a potential risk to the allergic child. This concern may be in the context of continued family consumption when the patient is allergic, or may be related to the recommendation that children at high risk for development of food allergy consume allergenic foods in a home with a nut-allergic sibling. Education about the routes of exposure that are necessary to produce a reaction and the ways of preparing food that prevent reactions is important to alleviate unnecessary fear.[31] Families should be counseled that having an allergy does not necessitate removal of a given food from the home. This decision must be made by the family considering their preferences.

OLDER CHILDREN WITH PEANUT ALLERGY

The case example presents the scenario of introducing tree nuts in a young child whose risk for preexisting tree nut allergy is lower than in older children.[7] Many older children with peanut allergy have been avoiding tree nuts either because of direct instructions not to eat them or they simply avoided them out of preference. If those patients and families want to introduce tree nuts, there is likely more risk for them to react. Again, there is no evidence or guidance about how to do this. In older children, prescreening with skin or blood testing before introduction should be considered. Providing the information that there is more risk in older children will allow the clinician and the family to make a more informed decision about testing before introduction. It remains necessary to have a similar discussion with the family about the characteristics of the testing, and what would be the next steps based on the results.

CASE UPDATE: FOLLOW-UP

Emily presents for follow-up 3 months after the initial visit. Her parents have introduced a variety of tree nuts without reaction, and she now enjoys mixed-nut butter a few times a week. They have continued to avoid peanut in all forms, and have no new food allergy concerns.

SUMMARY

Patients and families who experience a diagnosis of 1 nut allergy have a great deal to learn. Allergists must be a resource for the families to make informed decisions about the options for introducing nuts to which their children are not allergic. They can assist them in making a decision by understanding their preferences and goals. Whatever choice the family makes is the correct decision. Allergists need to allow families to make these decisions by having discussions with them before allergy testing to foods that have not caused a reaction. As new information in food allergy emerges, safe liberalization of the diets of a peanut-allergic or tree nut–allergic children to include other nuts should be offered.

REFERENCES

1. NIAID-Sponsored Expert Panel, Boyce JA, Assa'ad A, et al. Guidelines for the diagnosis and management of food allergy in the United States: report of the NIAID-sponsored expert panel. J Allergy Clin Immunol 2010;126(6 Suppl):S1–58.
2. Greenhawt M. Food allergy quality of life and living with food allergy. Curr Opin Allergy Clin Immunol 2016;16(3):284–90.
3. Sampson HA, Aceves S, Bock SA, et al. Food allergy: a practice parameter update 2014. J Allergy Clin Immunol 2014;134(5):1016–25.
4. Burks AW. Peanut allergy. Lancet 2008;371(9623):1538–46.

5. Sicherer SH, Sampson HA. Peanut allergy: emerging concepts and approaches for an apparent epidemic. J Allergy Clin Immunol 2007;120(3):491–503 [quiz: 504].
6. Couch C, Franxman T, Greenhawt M. Characteristics of tree nut challenges in tree nut allergic and tree nut sensitized individuals. Ann Allergy Asthma Immunol 2017;118(5):591–6.e3.
7. McWilliam V, Peters R, Tang MLK, et al. Patterns of tree nut sensitization and allergy in the first 6 years of life in a population-based cohort. J Allergy Clin Immunol 2018. https://doi.org/10.1016/j.jaci.2018.07.038.
8. Bird JA, Parrish C, Patel K, et al. Prevention of food allergy: beyond peanut. J Allergy Clin Immunol 2019. https://doi.org/10.1016/j.jaci.2018.12.993.
9. Brough HA, Turner PJ, Wright T, et al. Dietary management of peanut and tree nut allergy: what exactly should patients avoid? Clin Exp Allergy 2015;45(5):859–71.
10. Chan ES, Cummings C, Canadian Paediatric Society, Community Paediatrics Committee and Allergy Section. Dietary exposures and allergy prevention in high-risk infants: a joint statement with the Canadian Society of Allergy and Clinical Immunology. Paediatr Child Health 2013;18(10):545–54.
11. Du Toit G, Roberts G, Sayre PH, et al. Randomized trial of peanut consumption in infants at risk for peanut allergy. N Engl J Med 2015;372(9):803–13.
12. Ierodiakonou D, Garcia-Larsen V, Logan A, et al. Timing of allergenic food introduction to the infant diet and risk of allergic or autoimmune disease: a systematic review and meta-analysis. JAMA 2016;316(11):1181–92.
13. Perkin MR, Logan K, Tseng A, et al. Randomized trial of introduction of allergenic foods in breast-fed infants. N Engl J Med 2016;374(18):1733–43.
14. Peters RL, Neeland MR, Allen KJ. Primary prevention of food allergy. Curr Allergy Asthma Rep 2017;17(8):52.
15. Fleischer DM, Conover-Walker MK, Matsui EC, et al. The natural history of tree nut allergy. J Allergy Clin Immunol 2005;116(5):1087–93.
16. Windover AK, Boissy A, Rice TW, et al. The REDE model of healthcare communication: optimizing relationship as a therapeutic agent. J Patient Exp 2014; 1(1):8–13.
17. Togias A, Cooper SF, Acebal ML, et al. Addendum guidelines for the prevention of peanut allergy in the United States: report of the National Institute of Allergy and Infectious Diseases-sponsored expert panel. Ann Allergy Asthma Immunol 2017;118(2):166–73.e7.
18. Stiefel G, Anagnostou K, Boyle RJ, et al. BSACI guideline for the diagnosis and management of peanut and tree nut allergy. Clin Exp Allergy 2017;47(6):719–39.
19. Joshi PA, Smith J, Vale S, et al. The Australasian Society of Clinical Immunology and Allergy infant feeding for allergy prevention guidelines. Med J Aust 2019. https://doi.org/10.5694/mja2.12102.
20. Turner PJ, Campbell DE, Boyle RJ, et al. Primary prevention of food allergy: translating evidence from clinical trials to population-based recommendations. J Allergy Clin Immunol Pract 2018;6(2):367–75.
21. Koplin JJ, Peters RL, Dharmage SC, et al. Understanding the feasibility and implications of implementing early peanut introduction for prevention of peanut allergy. J Allergy Clin Immunol 2016;138(4):1131–41.e2.
22. Fisher HR, Keet CA, Lack G, et al. Preventing peanut allergy: where are we now? J Allergy Clin Immunol Pract 2019;7(2):367–73.
23. du Toit G, Sayre PH, Roberts G, et al. Allergen specificity of early peanut consumption and effect on development of allergic disease in the learning early about peanut allergy study cohort. J Allergy Clin Immunol 2018;141(4):1343–53.

24. Papadopoulos A, Elegbede CF, Ait-Dahmane S, et al. Tree nut allergy and anxiety related factors modulate food consumption behaviour in peanut-allergic patients: results of the MIRABEL survey. Regul Toxicol Pharmacol 2018;99:191–9.

25. Chan ES, Greenhawt MJ, Fleischer DM, et al. Managing cross-reactivity in those with peanut allergy. J Allergy Clin Immunol Pract 2018. https://doi.org/10.1016/j.jaip.2018.11.012.

26. Brough HA, Caubet J, Mazon A, et al. European Academy of Allergy and Clinical Immunology (EAACI) Congress 2017: Abstract 0124. Presented July 20, 2017. Allergy European Journal of Allergy and Clinical Immunology Volume 72, Issue S103 Special Issue: Abstracts from the European Academy of Allergy and Clinical Immunology Congress. Helsinki, Finland, June 17–21, 2017. p. 103–4.

27. Van Erp FC, Knulst AC, Kok IL, et al. Usefulness of open mixed nut challenges to exclude tree nut allergy in children. Clin Transl Allergy 2015;5:19.

28. Hostetler TL, Hostetler SG, Phillips G, et al. The ability of adults and children to visually identify peanuts and tree nuts. Ann Allergy Asthma Immunol 2012; 108(1):25–9.

29. Young I, Thaivalappil A. A systematic review and meta-regression of the knowledge, practices, and training of restaurant and food service personnel toward food allergies and Celiac disease. PLoS One 2018;13(9):e0203496.

30. McWilliam V, Koplin J, Lodge C, et al. The prevalence of tree nut allergy: a systematic review. Curr Allergy Asthma Rep 2015;15(9):54.

31. Sheehan WJ, Taylor SL, Phipatanakul W, et al. Environmental food exposure: what is the risk of clinical reactivity from cross-contact and what is the risk of sensitization. J Allergy Clin Immunol Pract 2018;6(6):1825–32.

Atopic Dermatitis Is a Barrier Issue, Not an Allergy Issue

Monica T. Kraft, MD[a], Benjamin T. Prince, MD, MSCI[a],*

KEYWORDS

- Atopic dermatitis • Eczema • Atopic march • Food allergy • Allergic rhinitis
- Asthma

KEY POINTS

- Atopic dermatitis is a chronic, relapsing, and pruritic disease that typically presents in early childhood and is the result of impaired epithelial barrier function and immunodysregulation.
- Allergen sensitization through the skin is likely an important initial step in the development of other allergic diseases in patients with atopic dermatitis.
- Although children with atopic dermatitis are more likely to produce specific Immunoglobulin E to both food and environmental allergens, there is conflicting evidence that allergen avoidance in these patients improves disease severity.
- The most effective treatments of atopic dermatitis are aimed at repairing and protecting the skin barrier and decreasing inflammation.

INTRODUCTION

Atopic dermatitis (AD) is a chronic, relapsing, and pruritic illness that affects up to 10% to 20% of children in developed countries and is associated with significant morbidity and decreased quality of life.[1] Within the United States, population studies have shown a national prevalence of 10.7% of children younger than 18 years, with a growing pool of evidence that the prevalence is increasing worldwide.[2]

Although the general term "eczema" was initially used to describe the condition, the correlation between eczema and other atopic conditions led to Wise and Sulzberger coining the term AD in 1933.[3] More recently, longitudinal studies have demonstrated that the presence of AD increases the risk of developing food allergy, allergic rhinitis, and asthma later in life.[4] This progression from AD to the manifestation of food allergy, allergic rhinitis, and asthma is often referred to the atopic march of childhood.

Disclosure Statement: Nothing to disclose.
[a] Department of Pediatrics, Division of Allergy and Immunology, Nationwide Children's Hospital, The Ohio State University College of Medicine, 700 Children's Drive, Columbus, OH 43205, USA
* Corresponding author.
E-mail address: benjamin.prince@nationwidechildrens.org

Although the exact cause of AD is not completely understood, it is thought to be the result of a complex interaction of genetic and environmental factors that ultimately leads to impaired epidermal barrier function and immune dysregulation. Because sensitization to environmental proteins often occurs as a result of a more porous skin barrier, it is a common misconception that allergy is at the root of the disease. In contrast, AD tends to be the initial manifestation of the atopic march, and sensitization through the skin is likely an important initial step in the development of other allergic diseases that have been associated with AD.[5]

This article reviews the clinical presentation, pathophysiology, and genetic factors associated with AD, briefly discusses proposed therapeutic strategies aimed at barrier repair, and describes the associations between AD and other allergic diseases.

CLINICAL PRESENTATION OF ATOPIC DERMATITIS
Clinical Features and Diagnosis

The characteristic features of AD are dry skin and severe pruritus. Although the clinical presentation can be variable, the disease typically begins in early childhood with a large proportion of cases going into remission during later childhood. Garmhausen and colleagues[6] analyzed more than 700 patients with AD and described 5 distinct subgroups based on symptom onset, disease course, and laboratory features. These investigators found that about one-third of all patients with AD had a disease history that began in early childhood and persisted until adulthood, and also noted that patients with early-onset AD were more likely to have other concomitant atopic conditions. Others have described 3 main age-related stages: infantile (up to age 2 years), childhood (ages 2–12 years), and adult.[7] The morphology of AD lesions varies with age. Infants tend to have red, crusted, and weeping patches located primarily on cheeks and extensor surfaces. Lesions become more papular in older children, localizing to flexural surfaces and often forming thickened, lichenified plaques. In adulthood, the disease can take on more of a relapsing and remitting course with flexures and hands continuing to be problem areas.[7]

Diagnosis is based on clinical history and the presence of characteristic eczematous lesions. Hanifin and Rajka[8] developed the initial diagnostic standard for AD in 1980, describing 4 major criteria and nearly 2 dozen minor criteria encompassing characteristics of the disease. Some of the minor criteria have been questioned since the initial publication because they are thought to not be specific to AD.[7] To remedy this, the United Kingdom Working Party attempted to refine the original Hanifin and Rajka criteria; however, their revision was not easily applied to young children.[9] In 2003, the American Academy of Dermatology (AAD) again revised the Hanifin and Rajka criteria to make it inclusive of all ages.[10] The AAD criteria are the most widely used in the United States and use essential characteristics of AD, important patient features, and less specific associated skin findings.

Natural History

AD follows a chronic or chronic-relapsing course over months to years, and the natural history of the disease is variable based on age of presentation and other clinical features. Although most patients will have resolution of AD by late childhood, in a proportion of cases the disease will persist into adulthood. Kim and colleagues[11] performed a meta-analysis of more than 45 studies including more than 110,000 subjects, and found that 80% of childhood AD did not persist past 8 years of age and a small percentage (less than 5%) persisted by more than 20 years after diagnosis. Another large longitudinal cohort study of more than 7000 patients showed that AD symptoms may persist longer than originally believed, as it was not until 20 years of age that 50% of patients reported at least one lifetime 6-month symptom-free and treatment-free period.[12] Peters and colleagues[13] performed a large prospective cohort study in Germany and found that genetic factors, early allergen sensitization, and a high-risk work environment were significant predictors of disease persistence through late adolescence.

PATHOPHYSIOLOGY OF ATOPIC DERMATITIS

Although food and environmental allergies are commonly implicated in the pathogenesis of AD, it is now well known that the disease is the result of skin barrier dysfunction and inappropriate immune response to skin antigens.[14]

Normal Skin Structure

The skin, specifically the epidermis, acts as a physical and immunologic protective barrier against the outside world. The epidermis is made up of keratinized stratified squamous epithelium in 4 main cell layers: the stratum basale, the stratum spinosum, the stratum granulosum, and the outermost layer, the stratum corneum.[15] The stratum corneum (made up of structural proteins, tight-junction proteins, ceramides, fatty acids, and cholesterol) is responsible for the primary barrier function of the epidermis. The stratum corneum itself is organized into 2 compartments, the corneocytes and the extracellular matrix, which prevent water loss and protect against microbial pathogens.[16] The structural makeup of the stratum corneum and the molecular organization of its multiple lipid bilayers creates the epidermis' permeable barrier. Absorption across the epidermis is primarily intercellular, through the lipid bilayer, and thus lipophilic molecules penetrate across the skin more readily than hydrophilic compounds.[17] Additional diffusion across the epidermis is accomplished paracellularly through tight-junction proteins that provide adhesive functions between keratinocytes.[14]

Structural Changes that Occur in Atopic Dermatitis

The main epithelial structural changes in AD that are thought to be responsible for disease pathogenesis include keratinocyte dysfunction and altered lipid composition, which lead to increased permeability of the stratum corneum and increased transepidermal water loss (**Box 1**).

Defects in terminal differentiation of keratinocytes have been identified in patients with AD through comparisons between skin lesions in patients with psoriasis, AD, and normal human skin. Ong and colleagues[18] compared skin biopsy specimens from patients with psoriasis, AD, and healthy controls and found that patients with AD had a deficiency in the expression of antimicrobial peptides (cathelicidins and β-defensins). This has been suggested as a contributing factor for the superimposed skin infections that are frequently seen in patients with AD. In addition, elevations in proteases have been described in acute flares of AD, which have been associated with impaired barrier function and reduced skin capacitance.[19]

Changes in the intercellular lipid composition and structure of the stratum corneum can also contribute to the increased skin permeability seen in AD. Ishikawa and colleagues[20] found that total levels of ceramides were significantly lower in the affected sites of patients with AD compared with normal skin sites in healthy individuals. Janssens and colleagues[21] found that ceramide chain length and lipid organization were directly correlated with the skin barrier defects in patients with AD, even in nonlesional skin.

Box 1
Pathogenic changes that lead to epithelial barrier dysfunction and immunodysregulation in atopic dermatitis

Epidermal Changes

- Defective terminal differentiation of keratinocytes
- Structural changes within the stratum corneum
- Increases in protease production
- Decreased amounts of ceramides with altered lipid composition
- Increased transepidermal water loss

Immunologic Changes

- Mechanical trauma–induced TSLP, IL-33, and IL-25 production
- Marked production of Th2 and Th22 cytokines
- Increased production of IL-31, leading to itch
- Abnormal signaling in pattern recognition receptor pathways
- Decreased production of antimicrobial peptides (defensins, cathelicidins)

Microbiome Changes

- Decreased bacterial diversity
- Increased colonization with toxin-producing strains of *S aureus*

Impairment of the stratum corneum results in an increase in transepidermal water loss (TEWL) or a decrease in water-holding ability (capacitance). Studies have shown significantly higher TEWL and lower capacitance in the lesional skin of patients with AD compared with normal controls.[22] Other studies have demonstrated similar findings of compromised skin barrier function and increased TEWL even in nonlesional skin of patients with AD.[23]

Immunologic Changes that Occur in Atopic Dermatitis

In addition to the dysfunction of the epidermal barrier in AD, research into the pathogenesis of AD has highlighted the role of immunologic pathways in cutaneous inflammation and barrier dysfunction (see **Box 1**).

Hyperinflammatory state of atopic dermatitis

In patients with AD, disruption of the skin barrier is associated with the release of proinflammatory cytokines that promote chemoattractants and adhesional molecules to recruit T cells to cutaneous sites. In response to mechanical trauma, epithelial cells release thymic stromal lymphopoietin (TSLP), interleukin (IL)-33, and IL-25.[24–26] This is associated with an increase in type 2 innate lymphoid cells (ILC2s) that drive the production of IL-5 and IL-13 and ultimately lead to T helper 2 (Th2) cell differentiation and inflammation. In addition to the inflammatory response produced by barrier disruption, others have reported on the increased expression of Th2, Th22, and Th1 cells in nonlesional skin of patients with AD compared with healthy subjects.[21] This finding suggests that systemic immune activation plays a role in the pathogenesis of eczema.

Immunologic changes in atopic dermatitis contribute to barrier dysfunction

In patients with AD, there is marked activation of Th2 and Th22 axes, causing profound increases in IL-4, IL-5, IL-13, IL-31, and IL-22.[27] These cytokines play a significant role in the pathogenesis of AD. IL-4 and IL-13 have been shown to affect keratinocyte differentiation, leading to a decreased expression of genes that are important for barrier function.[28] IL-22 acts synergistically with IL-17 to increase inflammation and contribute to barrier abnormalities.[29] IL-31 is thought to be responsible for the pathognomonic itch in eczema, and overexpression of IL-31 mRNA has been described in both lesional and nonlesional skin of patients with AD.[30] Subsequent scratching further disrupts the skin barrier, and the "itch-scratch" response has been shown in mouse models to enhance both Th1- and Th2-mediated inflammation.[31] Because of their role in the pathogenesis of AD, IL-4, IL-13, and IL-31 have subsequently become the targets of treatment with biological therapies.

Skin Microbiome Changes that Occur in Atopic Dermatitis

There is evidence that changes in the skin microbiome in patients with AD contribute to epithelial barrier dysfunction and exacerbate underlying immunodysregulation. Kong and colleagues[32] reported that skin bacterial diversity was decreased in AD compared with healthy controls. Patients with AD showed a greater proportion of *Staphylococcus* species (especially *Staphylococcus aureus*) during disease flares, with the presence of *S aureus* also being linked to increased disease severity. Other studies have identified *S aureus* colonization in greater than 90% of eczema lesions.[33] It is thought that the Th2 inflammation seen in AD facilitates *S aureus* binding by down-regulating keratinocyte production of antimicrobial peptides.[34] It has been shown that *S aureus* toxin production can lead to exacerbations in AD by causing regulatory T cell dysfunction and promoting inflammation.[35] Additionally *S aureus* can produce an extracellular protease, which has been suggested to disrupt the epidermal barrier.[36]

GENETIC CAUSES OF ATOPIC DERMATITIS

Studies of twin populations have historically demonstrated the heritability of AD.[37,38] Multiple genetic factors have been identified to be associated with the development of AD, with most genes playing a role in skin barrier integrity.

Genes Important for Skin Structure

Several of the genes that have been associated with the development of AD are located on chromosome 1q21 in an area termed the epidermal differentiation complex (EDC).[39] These genes code for proteins that are important for epithelial keratinocytes to produce the tough, cornified envelope of the epidermis that is integral for the barrier function. The strongest known genetic risk factors for AD are loss-of-function (LOF) mutations in the filaggrin gene *(FLG)*, which is located in the EDC.[40] *FLG* provides instructions for making the large protein called profilaggrin. Profilaggrin is ultimately cleaved to produce filaggrin, which is one of the final proteins necessary for the process of cornification. LOF mutations in *FLG* were first identified during studies investigating ichythyosis vulgaris, a disorder of keratinization and epidermal dysfunction.[41] Later studies have consistently demonstrated that LOF variants in filaggrin were also associated with AD.[42] The discovery of decreased filaggrin expression in patients with AD contributed significantly to the understanding of the pathogenesis of eczema. *FLG2* and *SPRR3* are 2 other genes located within the EDC that have been implicated in AD, both of which code for proteins that are important for the structure of the cornified envelope.[43]

Other genes not located within the EDC identified in patients with AD include *SPINK5*,[44] *CLDN1*,[45] and *TMEM79*.[46] All of these genes code for proteins that are important for epidermal homeostasis and barrier function.

THERAPEUTIC STRATEGIES OF BARRIER REPAIR IN ATOPIC DERMATITIS
Primary Prevention

There is evidence to support the proposal that the application of emollients early in life leads to a decreased incidence of AD. Because the stratum corneum is more permeable in infants younger than 1 year, it had been hypothesized that early emollient use could prevent AD in infants at risk for disease.[47] Horimukai and colleagues[48] performed the first randomized controlled trial of emollient use during the first months of life and found that approximately 32% fewer neonates developed AD in the treatment group. Although allergic sensitization was associated with eczematous skin, the study did not find a statistically significant effect of emollient use on the prevention of allergic sensitization as measured by allergen-specific immunoglobulin E (IgE). Simpson and colleagues[47] performed a randomized controlled trial evaluating emollient use in neonates at high risk for AD in the United States and United Kingdom. The investigators found that infants who used daily, full-body emollients had a relative risk reduction of 50% for incidence of AD at 6 months. Lowe and colleagues[49] evaluated emollient use in an Australian population of neonates and found that prophylactic emollient use for the first 6 months of life was associated with a trend toward reduced incidence of AD and food sensitization at both 6 and 12 months of age, although this study's results did not reach statistical significance.

Secondary and Tertiary Prevention

Cleansing and moisturization are the mainstay of treatment in AD, and current recommendations are for a short bath or shower followed immediately by the application of emollient moisturizer when the skin is still slightly wet.[50] This approach promotes improved hydration of the skin, whereas bathing alone without moisturization may result in decreased skin hydration. Adding diluted bleach to bathwater or other antiseptic cleansers provides antibacterial activity that can help in the management of AD given the increased colonization with S aureus and other pathogens.[51]

Emollients have remained a mainstay for the treatment of AD, providing a lipid-rich moisturizer that compensates for the lipid and ceramide deficiencies in AD skin.[50] In addition, studies have shown that aggressive emollient use as maintenance and prevention therapy in AD can reduce the number of prescriptions for topical corticosteroids and other medications in severe disease.[52] There is no single emollient that has emerged as the ideal maintenance therapy, and previous randomized controlled trials have shown similar efficacy for over-the-counter petroleum-based emollients and prescription barrier creams for monotherapy in AD.[53]

For more intensive moisture replacement, wet-wrap therapy can be used alone or in conjunction with topical steroids. This approach involves the application of a layer of wet cotton garments over topical treatment, and has been shown to improve AD severity and reduce the need for systemic immunosuppressive therapies.[54]

ASSOCIATION BETWEEN ATOPIC DERMATITIS AND ALLERGIC DISEASE
General Overview of the Atopic March and IgE-Mediated Disease

As previously discussed, the atopic march describes the typical progression of allergic diseases in childhood, with AD presenting early and food allergy, allergic rhinitis, and asthma presenting later. Proposed molecular mechanisms for the atopic march suggest that skin sensitization after allergen exposure induces local inflammation with Th2 cells that subsequently migrate through the blood to other sites including the respiratory mucosa of the lungs and nasal passages. Mouse models have shown that epicutaneous exposure to food protein antigens (such as ovalbumin and peanut protein) leads to Th2-mediated skin inflammation and a systemic immune response.[55] Using data from a cohort of preschool children with peanut allergy, Lack and colleagues[56] identified that the use of creams containing peanut oil during the first 6 months of life was significantly associated with increased risk for peanut allergy. Other studies have detected increased TEWL in the neonatal period in infants who later developed food allergy, further suggesting a link between skin barrier impairment and sensitization to food allergens.[57]

In studying the impact of AD on the manifestation of other allergic diseases, it is important to differentiate between sensitization, defined as the detection of IgE antibodies to a specific allergen through either serum or skin-prick testing (SPT), and the presence of clinical allergic disease. Many studies use environmental and food sensitization as an analog of allergic disease; however, the presence of allergen sensitization does not perfectly correlate with the presence of true allergy.

Atopic Dermatitis, Asthma, and Allergic Rhinitis

Atopic dermatitis is a risk factor for asthma and allergic rhinitis
Multiple birth cohort studies have described an association between early eczema and subsequent development of asthma. Horwood and colleagues[58] first identified early eczema as a risk factor for the development of asthma in a cohort of New Zealand children in their 1984 study. Subsequent cohort studies have also shown that early eczema was associated with increased risk of wheezing and asthma later in childhood.[59–61]

Studies of the German Multicenter Atopy Study cohort identified a significant association between AD and wheeze at age 7 years, but reported that most of these children also had documented wheezing in early childhood, which the authors argue is suggestive of a comanifesting disease process.[62] However, the Melbourne Atopic Cohort Study (MACS) showed that even after controlling for sensitization and early wheeze, AD was still significantly associated with an increased risk of asthma in boys.[63] More recently, data from the Canadian Healthy Infant Longitudinal Development Study found that AD without allergic sensitization was not associated with an increased risk of asthma.[4] The investigators argue that the combination of AD and allergic sensitization had interactive effects on asthma and food allergy risk. Additional studies of the MACS cohort have demonstrated that early-onset severe AD is most strongly associated with development of asthma and hay fever later in childhood.[64]

Environmental allergen avoidance strategies have shown limited improvement of atopic dermatitis
Despite the association between aeroallergens and AD, there is limited evidence to suggest that avoidance strategies improve AD severity. In several prospective, randomized controlled studies of avoidance strategies for house dust mite, there were no differences in sensitization to dust mite or incidence of AD when compared with those without avoidance strategies.[65–67] In fact, in 2 studies AD was more prevalent in the treatment group (ie, those using mattress covers to prevent dust mite exposure) compared with the control group.[67,68] In a Cochrane review including 7 studies of more than 300 children and adults with AD, the authors found mixed evidence regarding treatment response to dust mite avoidance in patients with AD.[69]

Atopic Dermatitis and Food Allergy

Atopic dermatitis increases the risk of food sensitization and allergy
There is evidence to support the notion that AD increases the risk of food sensitization. In the MACS, involving more than 600 infants, the presence of AD before 6 months of

age increased the risk of developing a new positive SPT result at 1 year.[70] In addition, early-onset persistent AD has been associated with allergic sensitization to food allergens within the first 2 years of life.[71] In a large Australian cohort study, up to 50% of patients with early-onset and severe AD had developed challenge-proven food allergy by 12 months of age, and overall infants with AD were approximately 5 times more likely to develop food allergy in comparison with infants without AD.[72]

As previously described, LOF mutations in *FLG* are an important part of the pathogenesis of skin barrier disruption in AD. Some studies have also reported an increased risk of food allergy in patients with LOF mutations in *FLG*.[73,74] However, others have shown that *FLG* mutations do not increase the risk of food allergy over and above that of food sensitization.[75]

Elimination diets in eczema have shown no prolonged benefit

Despite the association between early-onset severe AD and the prevalence of food allergy, it is noteworthy that studies evaluating elimination or exclusion diets as treatment of AD have not shown prolonged benefit.[76] An early study of avoidance of milk and egg in children with AD showed some improvement in pruritus and sleeplessness,[77] although a different study of milk- and egg-exclusion diets showed no significant benefit.[78] Whereas 2 studies showed a significant clinical improvement in SCORAD index for eczema severity in patients with cow's milk allergy/intolerance and AD after milk elimination,[79,80] pooled data in a comprehensive review including these studies found no difference in AD severity at 2 to 3 months or 6 to 8 months.[76] One study of children with egg sensitivity and AD did show some improvement in eczema severity score after egg elimination.[81] However, trials of elemental diets in adults and children with AD have not demonstrated improvement in AD symptoms or severity.[82,83] Lastly, a trial of a limited, few-foods diet in which all foods were excluded except for 5 to 8 failed to show benefit in AD symptoms or severity.[84]

Prolonged food avoidance may lead to immediate IgE-mediated reactions

With the growing evidence to support early introduction to prevent food allergy and the limited evidence to support elimination diets for the treatment of AD, it is important to be aware of the risks associated with elimination diets. There have been multiple case reports of patients on elimination diets for AD who previously tolerated the eliminated food developing acute allergic reactions after accidental ingestion or reintroduction of the food.[85–87] Furthermore, a retrospective chart review performed by Chang and colleagues[88] found that 19% of patients who had eliminated food for treatment of AD developed new, immediate allergic reactions after reintroduction to the food.

SUMMARY

AD is a chronic, relapsing disease that typically manifests in early childhood and improves with age in most individuals. It is the result of genetic and environmental factors that lead to impaired epidermal barrier function, increased TEWL, and immune dysregulation. Primary prevention strategies of replenishing epithelial water loss and maintaining the skin barrier early in life with daily emollient application have shown success. In patients with established AD, the most effective treatments are aimed at repairing and protecting the skin barrier and decreasing inflammation.

Many studies have demonstrated that AD is the start of an atopic march that leads to the development of other allergic diseases later in life, likely as a result of antigen exposure through a more porous and inflamed skin barrier. Although children with AD are more likely to produce specific IgE to both food and environmental allergens, there is conflicting evidence that allergen avoidance in these patients significantly improves disease severity. Furthermore, food-elimination diets in patients with AD may increase the risk of developing immediate, life-threatening reactions to the removed food. Given these findings, it is important to educate and counsel parents of children with AD about the disease pathogenesis, proven treatment strategies, and the limited benefit and even potential harm associated with strict allergen avoidance.

REFERENCES

1. Lyons JJ, Milner JD, Stone KD. Atopic dermatitis in children: clinical features, pathophysiology, and treatment. Immunol Allergy Clin North Am 2015;35:161–83.
2. Shaw TE, Currie GP, Koudelka CW, et al. Eczema prevalence in the United States: data from the 2003 National Survey of Children's Health. J Invest Dermatol 2011; 131:67–73.
3. Wise F, Sulzberger M. The 1933 year book of dermatology and syphilology. Chicago (IL): Year Book Publishers; 1934.
4. Tran MM, Lefebvre DL, Dharma C, et al. Predicting the atopic march: results from the Canadian Healthy Infant Longitudinal Development Study. J Allergy Clin Immunol 2018;141:601–7.e8.
5. Han H, Roan F, Ziegler SF. The atopic march: current insights into skin barrier dysfunction and epithelial cell-derived cytokines. Immunol Rev 2017;278:116–30.
6. Garmhausen D, Hagemann T, Bieber T, et al. Characterization of different courses of atopic dermatitis in adolescent and adult patients. Allergy 2013;68:498–506.
7. Rudikoff D, Lebwohl M. Atopic dermatitis. Lancet 1998;351:1715–21.
8. Hanifin JM, Rajka G. Diagnostic features of atopic dermatitis. Acta Derm Venereol 1980;92(Suppl):44–7.
9. Williams HC, Burney PG, Hay RJ, et al. The U.K. Working Party's diagnostic criteria for atopic dermatitis. I. Derivation of a minimum set of discriminators for atopic dermatitis. Br J Dermatol 1994;131:383–96.
10. Eichenfield LF, Tom WL, Chamlin SL, et al. Guidelines of care for the management of atopic dermatitis: section 1. Diagnosis and assessment of atopic dermatitis. J Am Acad Dermatol 2014;70:338–51.
11. Kim JP, Chao LX, Simpson EL, et al. Persistence of atopic dermatitis (AD): a systematic review and meta-analysis. J Am Acad Dermatol 2016;75:681–7.e11.
12. Margolis JS, Abuabara K, Bilker W, et al. Persistence of mild to moderate atopic dermatitis. JAMA Dermatol 2014;150:593–600.
13. Peters AS, Kellberger J, Vogelberg C, et al. Prediction of the incidence, recurrence, and persistence of atopic dermatitis in adolescence: a prospective cohort study. J Allergy Clin Immunol 2010;126:590–5.e1–3.
14. Weidinger S, Novak N. Atopic dermatitis. Lancet 2016;387:1109–22.
15. Matsui T, Amagai M. Dissecting the formation, structure and barrier function of the stratum corneum. Int Immunol 2015;27:269–80.
16. Elias PM. Stratum corneum defensive functions: an integrated view. J Invest Dermatol 2005;125:183–200.
17. Kezic S, Novak N, Jakasa I, et al. Skin barrier in atopic dermatitis. Front Biosci (Landmark Ed) 2014;19:542–56.
18. Ong PY, Ohtake T, Brandt C, et al. Endogenous antimicrobial peptides and skin infections in atopic dermatitis. N Engl J Med 2002;347:1151–60.
19. Voegeli R, Rawlings AV, Breternitz M, et al. Increased stratum corneum serine protease activity in acute eczematous atopic skin. Br J Dermatol 2009;161:70–7.

20. Ishikawa J, Narita H, Kondo N, et al. Changes in the ceramide profile of atopic dermatitis patients. J Invest Dermatol 2010;130:2511–4.

21. Janssens M, van Smeden J, Gooris GS, et al. Increase in short-chain ceramides correlates with an altered lipid organization and decreased barrier function in atopic eczema patients. J Lipid Res 2012;53:2755–66.

22. Holm EA, Wulf HC, Thomassen L, et al. Instrumental assessment of atopic eczema: validation of transepidermal water loss, stratum corneum hydration, erythema, scaling, and edema. J Am Acad Dermatol 2006;55:772–80.

23. Gupta J, Grube E, Ericksen MB, et al. Intrinsically defective skin barrier function in children with atopic dermatitis correlates with disease severity. J Allergy Clin Immunol 2008;121:725–30.e2.

24. Soumelis V, Reche PA, Kanzler H, et al. Human epithelial cells trigger dendritic cell mediated allergic inflammation by producing TSLP. Nat Immunol 2002;3: 673–80.

25. Savinko T, Matikainen S, Saarialho-Kere U, et al. IL-33 and ST2 in atopic dermatitis: expression profiles and modulation by triggering factors. J Invest Dermatol 2012;132:1392–400.

26. Wang YH, Angkasekwinai P, Lu N, et al. IL-25 augments type 2 immune responses by enhancing the expansion and functions of TSLP-DC-activated Th2 memory cells. J Exp Med 2007;204:1837–47.

27. Czarnowicki T, Krueger JG, Guttman-Yassky E. Skin barrier and immune dysregulation in atopic dermatitis: an evolving story with important clinical implications. J Allergy Clin Immunol Pract 2014;2:371–9.

28. Howell MD, Kim BE, Gao P, et al. Cytokine modulation of atopic dermatitis filaggrin skin expression. J Allergy Clin Immunol 2007;120:150–5.

29. Gittler JK, Shemer A, Suárez-Fariñas M, et al. Progressive activation of T(H)2/T(H) 22 cytokines and selective epidermal proteins characterizes acute and chronic atopic dermatitis. J Allergy Clin Immunol 2012;130:1344–54.

30. Kato A, Fujii E, Watanabe T, et al. Distribution of IL-31 and its receptor expressing cells in skin of atopic dermatitis. J Dermatol Sci 2014;74:229–35.

31. Mihara K, Kuratani K, Matsui T, et al. Vital role of the itch-scratch response in development of spontaneous dermatitis in NC/Nga mice. Br J Dermatol 2004; 151:335–45.

32. Kong HH, Oh J, Deming C, et al. Temporal shifts in the skin microbiome associated with disease flares and treatment in children with atopic dermatitis. Genome Res 2012;22:850–9.

33. Aly R, Maibach HI, Shinefield HR. Microbial flora of atopic dermatitis. Arch Dermatol 1977;113:780–2.

34. Brauweiler AM, Goleva E, Leung DY. Th2 cytokines increase *Staphylococcus aureus* alpha toxin- induced keratinocyte death through the signal transducer and activator of transcription 6 (STAT6). J Invest Dermatol 2014;134:2114–21.

35. Ou L-S, Goleva E, Hall C, et al. T regulatory cells in atopic dermatitis and subversion of their activity by superantigens. J Allergy Clin Immunol 2004;113(4): 756–63.

36. Hirasawa Y, Takai T, Nakamura T, et al. *Staphylococcus aureus* extracellular protease causes epidermal barrier dysfunction. J Invest Dermatol 2010;130:614–7.

37. Schultz Larsen F. Atopic dermatitis: a genetic-epidemiologic study in a population-based twin sample. J Am Acad Dermatol 1993;28:719–23.

38. Thomsen SF, Ulrik CS, Kyvik KO, et al. Importance of genetic factors in the etiology of atopic dermatitis: a twin study. Allergy Asthma Proc 2007;28:535–9.

39. Mischke D, Korge BP, Marenholz I, et al. Genes encoding structural proteins of epidermal cornification and S100 calcium-binding proteins form a gene complex ('epidermal differentiation complex') on human chromosome 1q21. J Invest Dermatol 1996;106:989–92.

40. Irvine AD, McLean WHI, Leung DYM. Filaggrin mutations associated with skin and allergic diseases. N Engl J Med 2011;365:1315–27.

41. Smith FJD, Irvine AD, Terron-Kwiatkowski A, et al. Loss-of-function mutations in the gene encoding filaggrin cause ichthyosis vulgaris. Nat Genet 2006;38: 337–42.

42. Palmer CNA, Irvine AD, Terron-Kwiatkowski A, et al. Common loss-of-function variants of the epidermal barrier protein filaggrin are a major predisposing factor for atopic dermatitis. Nat Genet 2006;38:441–6.

43. Marenholz I, Rivera VA, Esparza-Gordillo J, et al. Association screening in the Epidermal Differentiation Complex (EDC) identifies an SPRR3 repeat number variant as a risk factor for eczema. J Invest Dermatol 2011;131:1644–9.

44. Kato A, Fukai K, Oiso N, et al. Association of SPINK5 gene polymorphisms with atopic dermatitis in the Japanese population. Br J Dermatol 2003;148:665–9.

45. De Benedetto A, Rafaels NM, McGirt LY, et al. Tight junction defects in patients with atopic dermatitis. J Allergy Clin Immunol 2011;127:773–86.e1–7.

46. Saunders SP, Goh CS, Brown SJ, et al. Tmem79/Matt is the matted mouse gene and is a predisposing gene for atopic dermatitis in human subjects. J Allergy Clin Immunol 2013;132:1121–9.

47. Simpson EL, Berry TM, Brown PA, et al. A pilot study of emollient therapy for the primary prevention of atopic dermatitis. J Am Acad Dermatol 2010;63:587–93.

48. Horimukai K, Morita K, Narita M, et al. Application of moisturizer to neonates prevents development of atopic dermatitis. J Allergy Clin Immunol 2014;134: 824–30.e6.

49. Lowe AJ, Su JC, Allen KJ, et al. A randomized trial of a barrier lipid replacement strategy for the prevention of atopic dermatitis and allergic sensitization: the PEBBLES pilot study. Br J Dermatol 2018;178:e19–21.

50. Wollenberg A, Szepietowski J, Taieb A, et al. Consensus-based European guidelines for treatment of atopic eczema (atopic dermatitis) in adults and children: part I. J Eur Acad Dermatol Venereol 2018;32:657–82.

51. Wong S, Ng TG, Baba R. Efficacy and safety of sodium hypochlorite (bleach) baths in patients with moderate to severe atopic dermatitis in Malaysia. J Dermatol 2013;40:874–80.

52. Grimalt R, Mengeaud V, Cambazard F, Study Investigators' Group.. The steroid-sparing effect of an emollient therapy in infants with atopic dermatitis: a randomized controlled study. Dermatology 2007;214:61–7.

53. Miller DW, Koch SB, Yentzer BA, et al. An over-the-counter moisturizer is as clinically effective as, and more cost-effective than, prescription barrier creams in the treatment of children with mild-to-moderate atopic dermatitis: a randomized, controlled trial. J Drugs Dermatol 2011;10:531–7.

54. González-López G, Ceballos-Rodríguez RM, González-López JJ, et al. Efficacy and safety of wet wrap therapy for patients with atopic dermatitis: a systematic review and meta-analysis. Br J Dermatol 2017;177:688–95.

55. Strid J, Hourihane J, Kimber I, et al. Disruption of the stratum corneum allows potent epicutaneous immunization with protein antigens resulting in a dominant systemic Th2 response. Eur J Immunol 2004;34:2100–9.

56. Lack G, Fox D, Northstone K, et al. Factors associated with the development of peanut allergy in childhood. N Engl J Med 2003;348:977–85.

57. Kelleher MM, Dunn-Galvin A, Gray C, et al. Skin barrier impairment at birth predicts food allergy at 2 years of age. J Allergy Clin Immunol 2016;137:1111–6.e8.
58. Horwood LJ, Fergusson DM, Shannon FT. Social and familial factors in the development of early childhood asthma. Pediatrics 1985;75:859–68.
59. Arshad SH, Kurukulaaratchy RJ, Fenn M, et al. Early life risk factors for current wheeze, asthma, and bronchial hyperresponsiveness at 10 years of age. Chest 2005;127:502–8.
60. Saunes M, Øien T, Dotterud CK, et al. Early eczema and the risk of childhood asthma: a prospective, population-based study. BMC Pediatr 2012;12:168.
61. von Kobyletzki LB, Bornehag CG, Hasselgren M, et al. Eczema in early childhood is strongly associated with the development of asthma and rhinitis in a prospective cohort. BMC Dermatol 2012;12:11.
62. Illi S, von Mutius E, Lau S, et al. The natural course of atopic dermatitis from birth to age 7 years and the association with asthma. J Allergy Clin Immunol 2004;113: 925–31.
63. Lowe AJ, Carlin JB, Bennett CM, et al. Do boys do the atopic march while girls dawdle? J Allergy Clin Immunol 2008;121:1190–5.
64. Lowe AJ, Angelica B, Su J, et al. Age at onset and persistence of eczema are related to subsequent risk of asthma and hay fever from birth to 18 years of age. Pediatr Allergy Immunol 2017;28:384–90.
65. Custovic A, Simpson BM, Simpson A, et al. Effect of environmental manipulation in pregnancy and early life on respiratory symptoms and atopy during first year of life: a randomised trial. Lancet 2001;358:188–93.
66. Horak F, Matthews S, Ihorst G, et al. Effect of mite-impermeable mattress encasings and an educational package on the development of allergies in a multinational randomized, controlled birth-cohort study—24 months results of the Study of Prevention of Allergy in Children in Europe. Clin Exp Allergy 2004;34: 1220–5.
67. Koopman LP, van Strien RT, Kerkhof M, et al. Placebo-controlled trial of house dust mite-impermeable mattress covers: effect on symptoms in early childhood. Am J Respir Crit Care Med 2002;166:307–13.
68. Mihrshahi S, Peat JK, Marks GB, et al. Eighteen-month outcomes of house dust mite avoidance and dietary fatty acid modification in the Childhood Asthma Prevention Study (CAPS). J Allergy Clin Immunol 2003;111:162–8.
69. Nankervis H, Pynn EV, Boyle RJ, et al. House dust mite reduction and avoidance measures for treating eczema. Cochrane Database Syst Rev 2015;(1):CD008426. https://doi.org/10.1002/14651858.CD008426.pub2.
70. Lowe AJ, Abramson MJ, Hosking CS, et al. The temporal sequence of allergic sensitization and onset of infantile eczema. Clin Exp Allergy 2007;37:536–42.
71. Carlsten C, Dimich-Ward H, Ferguson A, et al. Atopic dermatitis in a high-risk cohort: natural history, associated allergic outcomes, and risk factors. Ann Allergy Asthma Immunol 2013;110:24–8.
72. Martin PE, Eckert JK, Koplin JJ, et al. Which infants with eczema are at risk of food allergy? Results from a population-based cohort. Clin Exp Allergy 2015; 45:255–64.
73. Brown SJ, Asai Y, Cordell HJ, et al. Loss-of-function variants in the filaggrin gene are a significant risk factor for peanut allergy. J Allergy Clin Immunol 2011;127: 661–7.
74. Venkataraman D, Soto-Ramírez N, Kurukulaaratchy RJ, et al. Filaggrin loss-of-function mutations are associated with food allergy in childhood and adolescence. J Allergy Clin Immunol 2014;134:876–82.e4.

75. Tan H-TT, Ellis JA, Koplin JJ, et al. Filaggrin loss-of-function mutations do not predict food allergy over and above the risk of food sensitization among infants. J Allergy Clin Immunol 2012;130:1211–3.e3.
76. Bath-Hextall F, Delamere FM, Williams HC. Dietary exclusions for improving established atopic eczema in adults and children: systematic review. Allergy 2009;64:258–64.
77. Atherton DJ, Sewell M, Soothill JF, et al. A double-blind controlled crossover trial of an antigen-avoidance diet in atopic eczema. Lancet 1978;1:401–3.
78. Neild VS, Marsden RA, Bailes JA, et al. Egg and milk exclusion diets in atopic eczema. Br J Dermatol 1986;114:117–23.
79. Niggemann B, Binder C, Dupont C, et al. Prospective, controlled, multi-center study on the effect of an amino-acid-based formula in infants with cow's milk allergy/intolerance and atopic dermatitis. Pediatr Allergy Immunol 2001;12:78–82.
80. Isolauri E, Sütas Y, Mäkinen-Kiljunen S, et al. Efficacy and safety of hydrolyzed cow milk and amino acid-derived formulas in infants with cow milk allergy. J Pediatr 1995;127:550–7.
81. Lever R, MacDonald C, Waugh P, et al. Randomised controlled trial of advice on an egg exclusion diet in young children with atopic eczema and sensitivity to eggs. Pediatr Allergy Immunol 1998;9:13–9.
82. Munkvad M, Danielsen L, Høj L, et al. Antigen-free diet in adult patients with atopic dermatitis. A double-blind controlled study. Acta Derm Venereol 1984;64:524–8.
83. Leung TF, Ma KC, Cheung LT, et al. A randomized, single-blind and crossover study of an amino acid-based milk formula in treating young children with atopic dermatitis. Pediatr Allergy Immunol 2004;15:558–61.
84. Mabin DC, Sykes AE, David TJ. Controlled trial of a few foods diet in severe atopic dermatitis. Arch Dis Child 1995;73:202–7.
85. Flinterman AE, Knulst AC, Meijer Y, et al. Acute allergic reactions in children with AEDS after prolonged cow's milk elimination diets. Allergy 2006;61:370–4.
86. David TJ. Anaphylactic shock during elimination diets for severe atopic eczema. Arch Dis Child 1984;59:983–6.
87. Barbi E, Gerarduzzi T, Longo G, et al. Fatal allergy as a possible consequence of long-term elimination diet. Allergy 2004;59:668–9.
88. Chang A, Robison R, Cai M, et al. Natural history of food-triggered atopic dermatitis and development of immediate reactions in children. J Allergy Clin Immunol Pract 2016;4:229–36.e1.

Tips and Tricks for Controlling Eczema

Rekha Raveendran, MD*

KEYWORDS

- Eczema • Dupilumab • Topical corticosteroids • Immunosuppressants
- Topical calcineurin inhibitors • Moisturizers

KEY POINTS

- Eczema is a chronic, relapsing, and remitting disease that requires daily skin care to prevent transepidermal water loss.
- Topical therapies are the preferred first step for treatment of eczema.
- Biological therapies are promising targeted treatment options for patients with moderate to severe eczema.
- For patients with recalcitrant eczema, it is important to rule out other diagnoses that may mimic the appearance of eczema.

INTRODUCTION

Eczema is a chronic inflammatory skin condition that affects 10% to 30% of children and is secondary to an impaired skin barrier.[1,2] This disease typically presents between birth and 5 years of age, and although most patients have resolution by adolescence, 10% to 20% can persist into adulthood.[2] Eczema, also commonly known as atopic dermatitis, is often the first sign of atopy and is associated with other atopic diseases including asthma, allergic rhinitis, and food allergy. The relapsing and remitting nature of eczema can make it difficult to control flare-ups. This article discusses different ways to help manage eczema and flare-ups.

SYMPTOMS

Impaired skin barrier function leads to increased transepidermal water loss, which ultimately leads to the presence of eczematous lesions. The presentation of eczematous lesions differs based on chronicity and age. Acute lesions can present with erythema,

Disclosure Statement: The author has no financial disclosures.
Division of Allergy/Immunology, Department of Otolaryngology, The Ohio State University Wexner Medical Center, OSU Eye and Ear Institute, 915 Olentangy River Road, Suite 4000, Columbus, OH 43212, USA
* 300 West Spring Street Unit 205, Columbus, OH 43215.
E-mail address: Rekha.Raveendran@osumc.edu

papules, vesicles, and occasionally serous exudate, whereas chronic ones can present with lichenification and hyperpigmentation.

In infancy and early childhood, typical lesions will be found on head, neck, and extensor surfaces. In adolescence and adulthood, however, the distribution is mainly on the flexural surfaces. There may also be distribution on the palms, soles, head, and neck. Eczema typically spares moist areas of the body, including the groin and axillary regions.[3]

DIAGNOSTIC TEST/IMAGING STUDY

Diagnosis of eczema is a clinical diagnosis, and there have been many different sets of proposed criterion over time. Hanifin and Rajka were the first to put together diagnostic criteria for eczema in 1980, with pruritus, relapsing nature, distribution, and atopy being identified as being major features along with several minor features. There have been many other iterations of proposed criterion, with the American Academy of Dermatology being the most used in the United States.[4]

In addition to physical features of eczema, there are also proposed scoring systems to determine severity of disease. This is important to differentiate because treatment options vary based on severity. The SCORing Atopic Dermatitis (SCORAD) is a commonly used tool to score severity. The SCORAD uses both objective measures of disease (body surface area affected and clinical features) along with the patient's subjective symptoms of itch and sleeplessness.[5] The objective measures are based on the expertise of the interpreting physician, and the subjective symptoms are based on the patient's perception, which gives a fully encompassing picture of the extent of disease and its impact on quality of life.

DIFFERENTIAL DIAGNOSIS

Conditions can mimic or overlap with eczema that can make it difficult to discern the underlying cause (**Table 1**). Severe eczema in infancy, especially those refractory to treatment, should be evaluated for possible underlying immunodeficiency. These

Table 1
Eczema mimics

Examples of Similarly Presenting Diseases	Associated Signs and Symptoms	Typical Time of Presentation
Immunodeficiency: Netherton syndrome Wiskott-Aldrich DOCK8 Hyper IgE syndrome	All: Failure to thrive Recurrent infections Eczema that recalcitrant to topical therapies	Infancy
Inflammatory diseases: Psoriasis Viral exanthem Contact dermatitis	Thickened plaques with silvery scale Morbilliform rash Pruritic, vesicular, in area of contact	Mainly in adolescence to adulthood Viral exanthems can present in infancy
Malignancy: Cutaneous T-cell lymphoma	Patchy eczematous rash Recalcitrant to topical steroids	Adulthood
Nutritional deficiency: Biotin Zinc	Failure to thrive Weight loss	Infancy/early childhood

patients tend to present with other associated symptoms including failure to thrive and recurrent infections. Inflammatory conditions such as seborrheic dermatitis, contact dermatitis, and nummular dermatitis often present with erythematous, scaling, pruritic rashes that are commonly mistaken for eczema. Infectious conditions such as impetigo present with crusting and irritation and may be secondary to complications from eczema. Lastly, in endemic areas of the world, nutritional deficiencies of zinc or biotin can lead to a dry, pruritic rash that is similar to eczema.[6] There are many rashes that can present similarly to eczema, and therefore it is important to differentiate between these conditions in order to provide optimal treatment.

TREATMENT
Nonpharmacologic Treatments

Dry skin care
The cornerstone of eczema treatment is prevention of transepidermal water loss. Because of the dysfunctional skin barrier, water loss is a chronic issue and requires daily skin care. Soaking baths in lukewarm water should be done at least once a day and should last about 10 minutes. Soaps should be bland and not contain any dyes or fragrances to avoid skin irritation. After bathing, the skin should be patted dry, allowing some moisture from the bath to remain on the surface, and should be immediately followed by application of moisturizer. The moisturizer will act as a sealant to lock in the moisture from the bath and will help keep the skin hydrated as well as restore the epidermal barrier.

Moisturizers
There are many different types of moisturizers available, including emollients, occlusive, and humectants (**Table 2**).

Emollients
The most commonly used moisturizers are emollients, which are used to soften the skin. Although emollients include both creams and lotions, cream-based emollients are preferred. Lotions contain higher percentage of water that is adequate for normal skin barriers. In eczematous skin, however, an impaired skin barrier leads to evaporation of the water-based lotion, leading to a paradoxic drying effect. Lotions are reserved for use on areas where there is less concern for water loss. Cream-based emollients, however, have a hydrophobic oil base that prevents rapid evaporation.[7]

There are many types of emollients on the market and they use a variety of additives to help bolster therapeutic efficacy. Prescription and over-the-counter preparations are available, but there have not been any studies to show that one preparation is more effective than another.

Occlusives
Ointments have higher lipid content than creams and provide an occlusive barrier. This may make ointments effective moisturizers. These formulations are generally greasier, however, which can make them more difficult to deal with and can lead to folliculitis or acne on more sensitive skin. Although they can be used on open skin without significant irritation or burning, patients may develop a contact reaction to ingredients such as lanolin, which can lead to worsening of eczema.[3,7,8]

Humectants
Humectants contain ingredients that help draw water toward itself and when used on the skin, will help hydrate the stratum corneum. Urea, lactic acid, and hyaluronic acid are the most commonly used humectants. They are effective moisturizers and can be

Table 2
Different types of moisturizers

Type of Moisturizer	Mode of Action	Common Additives	Advantages	Disadvantages
Emollients	Oil in water emulsion that fills in cracks of skin with oil leading to smoothing and softening of skin	Ceramides Cholesterol	Many options to choose from Smoothes over skin Softens skin	May not provide enough moisturization for severely dry skin Irritation or burning sensation with certain preparations
Occlusives	Hydrophobic barrier over skin to prevent transepidermal water loss	Lanolin Mineral oil Petrolatum Dimethicone	Provides thick layer to prevent water loss and can be very effective for severely dry skin	Greasy Can block follicles Can lead to contact dermatitis (lanolin)
Humectants	Attract water to itself, leading to hydration of the stratum corneum	Lactic acid Urea Glycerol	Can be very hydrating to dry skin	Can cause burning sensation on open skin

used on severely dry skin. They can cause a burning sensation on open skin, which may prohibit use and should mainly be used on intact skin.[3,7,8]

Bleach baths

Staphylococcus aureus colonization can lead to worsening of skin lesions and also superinfection. Dilute bleach baths have been used to decrease colonization of both lesional and nonlesional skin. These baths are cost-effective and generally well tolerated and have been recommended for use in eczema skin care. Recent studies, however, have reviewed the studies on bleach baths and although they do decrease colonization, there does not seem to be any advantage to the use of bleach over plain water baths.[9,10]

Wet wrap therapy

For patients with moderate to severe eczema the use of emollients and other topical therapies may not provide adequate relief. Wet wrap therapy is an affordable treatment that can be efficacious in refractory cases. In this therapy the patient soaks in warm water before patting dry. Application of an emollient is placed on skin followed by application of wet dressings on the affected areas. A dry dressing is placed over the wet dressing and is left in place for up to 24 hours. Dressings should be made of nonirritating, breathable fabric such as gauze or cotton. If full body treatment is needed, long underwear can be used as surrogate for wraps.[11] Use of topical corticosteroids in addition to wet wrap therapy has been shown not only to be efficacious but also works faster than wet wrap therapy with emollients alone.[12]

Although wet wrap therapy offers many advantages, particularly in moderate to severe eczema, it can be cumbersome. This does require time and cooperation from the patient and can be uncomfortable. Therefore, this therapy may be best used on those with difficult-to-treat eczema rather than a first-line therapy.

Irritant avoidance

Patients with eczema are at risk of developing other atopic diseases, including food allergy, asthma, and allergic rhinitis. The abnormal skin barrier increases sensitization to food, environmental, and contact allergens. Exposure to these irritants can lead to flares.

Food allergens

Eczema has been associated with food allergen sensitization that can result in different reactions. The most concerning reaction is an immediate immunoglobulin E (IgE)-mediated reaction leading to anaphylaxis. In these patients, allergy testing and strict avoidance of the implicated food is the standard treatment. Some patients, however, do not experience an immediate reaction and instead have a delayed eczematous flare in response to food ingestion. There have been several studies that have looked at patients with elevated IgE/IgE sensitization to foods. Patients with moderate to severe eczema tended to show improvement in their skin with elimination of the identified food trigger.[13–15] This correlation between foods and eczematous flares is mainly seen in the pediatric population and does not seem to extend to the adult population.[15]

Although there has been evidence of improvement with elimination diets in patients with IgE-mediated sensitization to foods and delayed eczematous flares, there is concern for possible risks associated with food elimination. Removing foods that contain nutrients important for growth, such as protein and calcium, from the diet can lead to nutritional deficiencies and growth retardation.[15] If foods are removed from the diet, it is important to ensure that the patient is getting appropriate supplementation and maintaining on their growth curve. Recent data have also shown that up to 19% to 83% of patients sensitized to foods without a previous history of immediate IgE-mediated reactions can develop them after a period of elimination.[15,16] It is therefore important to exercise caution and balance the risks and benefits before proceeding with allergy testing and elimination diets.

Aeroallergens
Contact reactions from aeroallergens have been associated in patients with eczema. Lesions tend to be on exposed areas of the body such as the neck and face. Dust mite has been the most implicated aeroallergen, with positive patch tests in up to 40% of patients.[17] Studies on dust mite avoidance, however, have shown conflicting results. One study showed that instituting several dust mite avoidance measures (dust mite encasings, vacuuming, and acaricides) showed significant improvement in eczema severity in comparison to placebo.[18] Other studies looking at dust mite encasements alone did show decrease in levels of dust mite antigen but did not see a significant improvement in eczema.[19] Other allergens have been implicated, including pet dander, cockroach, and pollens. The evidence on the efficacy of allergy immunotherapy has been mixed.[20]

Other irritants
Contact dermatitis is a type IV hypersensitivity reaction that can occur in conjunction with eczema. It is unclear, however, what the true prevalence is with reports varying between 27% and 95.6%.[21] Lanolin, metals, antibiotics, and fragrances are commonly associated contact allergens identified in those with eczema.[22] These contact allergens can be found in topical products including emollients and antimicrobials that are used to treat eczema, which can lead to paradoxic worsening. Patch testing is the gold standard to diagnose contact dermatitis and should be considered in patients who have persistent symptoms or worsening after treatment.

Pharmacologic Therapies

Topical corticosteroids
Topical corticosteroids (TCS) are considered first-line therapy for eczema. There are many different formulations and potencies that allow treatment to be tailored to severity and location (**Table 3**). Topical steroid potency ranges from low potency (Class 7) to super potency (Class 1), and they can be used for both acute and chronic management of eczema. Mild eczema and thinner-skinned areas, such as eyelids and face, should be treated with lower potency TCS to minimize potential side effects. More severe eczema and lichenified lesions, however, may require much stronger formulations to improve skin conditions.

In addition to potency of TCS, the amount of medication is also an important measure to be aware of. This, similar to potency, depends on the area of the body that is being treated. The finger-tip unit was first described in 1991 by Long and Finlay[23] as a practical measurement of topical therapies. It is described as the amount of ointment expressed from a tube with 5-mm diameter nozzle applied from the distal skin crease to the tip of the index finger. This amount varies slightly from men to women (0.49 g in men and 0.43 g in women) and covers 257 to 312 cm² of skin area.

TCS therapy is used in addition to daily skin care and should not be used as a replacement for moisturizing. Appropriate therapy generally requires twice daily application to the affected areas until the skin is clear. In patients with frequently relapsing eczema, TCS can be used as maintenance therapy in addition to the acute treatment. Application of low or medium potency TCS at commonly affected sites twice weekly has been shown to decrease flares.[7]

| Table 3 |
| Steroid potency ranges of topical corticosteroids |

Steroid Potency	Examples	Location of Use	Eczema Severity
Class 7: Least potent	Hydrocortisone cream 1%	Face Thinner-skinned	Mild
Class 6: Mild	Desonide cream 0.05% Hydrocortisone cream 2.5% Betamethasone valerate lotion 0.1% Fluocinolone acetonide oil 0.01%	areas of body such as eyelids Scalp	
Class 5: Lower Mid- Strength	Fluticasone propionate cream 0.05% Desonide ointment 0.05% Hydrocortisone valerate cream 0.2% Betamethasone valerate ointment 0.1%	Use on trunk and extremities Avoid thinner- skinned areas and face	Mild Moderate
Class 4: Mid-Strength	Triamcinolone acetonide cream 0.1% Mometasone furoate cream 0.1%		Moderate
Class 3: Upper Mid- Strength	Fluticasone propionate ointment 0.05% Desoximetasone cream 0.05% Betamethasone ointment 0.1% Fluocinonide cream 0.05%	Use: Trunk Extremities Palms Soles	Moderate to severe
Class 2: Potent	Mometasone furoate ointment 0.1% Fluocinonide ointment 0.05%	Lichenified areas Avoid: Face	Severe
Class 1: Superpotent	Clobetasol propionate cream 0.05% Betamethasone dipropionate ointment 0.05%	Thinner-skinned areas	Reserve use for severe eczema

Overall TCS are generally well tolerated, affordable, and effective, making them the ideal choice for first-line therapy. Potential adverse effects from TCS can occur, however, and include hypopigmentation, striae, acne, and skin atrophy. Choosing the appropriate strength and amount for the affected area can minimize these side effects.

Topical calcineurin inhibitors

Topical calcineurin inhibitors (TCIs) are a nonsteroidal topical therapy option for eczema. Currently there are 2 TCI options available in the United States. Pimecrolimus is available as a 1% cream and tacrolimus is available in both 0.1% and 0.03% ointment. Tacrolimus 0.1% is not approved for patients younger than 15 years, whereas the 0.03% ointment is approved for those from age 2 to 15 years.

TCIs can be used, similarly to TCS, for both acute and maintenance therapies. Treatment is usually twice daily on the affected area until the skin clears and can also be used prophylactically twice weekly to prevent flares. The finger-tip unit also applies to use of TCIs. Unlike TCS, however, TCIs do not cause skin atrophy and may be preferred for more delicate, thinner-skinned areas such as eyelids. For patients with severe eczema and large body surface area affected, there may be concern about systemic absorption of TCS. TCIs are a good alternative for these patients or can be used adjunctively on portions of the body as a steroid-sparing agent.

Major adverse effect with TCIs are burning and stinging and this is more noticeable on open, inflamed areas, which can preclude use if the patient is unable to tolerate this. The burning sensation tends to dissipate with consistent use and can be ameliorated by using a TCS on the area before using TCI or by placing the medication in the fridge before use.[7] TCIs do not have as many options as TCS; therefore, insurance coverage, availability, as well as cost may also be prohibitive for patients.

Crisaborole
More targeted topical therapies have recently been approved. Crisaborole is an anti-phosphodiesterase-4 (PDE4) inhibitor. PDE4 is an enzyme that is preferentially expressed in inflammatory cells. Anti-PDE4 oral therapies have been used in other dermatologic conditions such as psoriasis but were associated with gastrointestinal (GI) side effects.[24] Crisaborole is the first anti-PDE4 topical therapy available and has shown positive effects in 2 large-scale double-blinded studies. There was a greater percentage of clearing of eczema in the crisaborole arm than those with placebo vehicle ointment.[25] There were, however, many patients in the placebo arm who also had improvement in their symptoms, which may demonstrate the efficacy of the vehicle used in both arms in addition to the crisaborole.[24,25]

Crisaborole provides another topical nonsteroidal option for pediatric patients in addition to TCIs. Similar to TCIs, the major side effects are irritation, burning, and stinging at the site of application.

Antimicrobials/antifungals
The microbiome of eczematous lesions can vary with age. S aureus is found in 70% of eczematous lesions and 39% of unaffected skin in patients with eczema.[26] It can produce toxins that can lead to worsening inflammation and pruritus leading to worsening flares. Topical mupirocin or oral antibiotics can be used in patients with crusting and superinfected flares. For adolescents and adults, head and neck atopic dermatitis can be colonized with fungi. Malassezia furfur is the most implicated organism.[27] Azole antifungals, particularly topical ketoconazole, can be used to decrease flares in those who are colonized with M furfur. Use of antimicrobial or antifungal therapy can be a good adjunctive treatment in patients with difficult-to-control flares.

Systemic Therapy

Oral steroids
Oral corticosteroids are potent antiinflammatory medications and can provide rapid improvement to severe and persistent eczema. Because of the quick resolution with oral steroids, they are frequently prescribed and are often preferred by patients. Unfortunately, oral steroids can cause a rebound effect with worsening flares after the course of steroids is finished, which can lead to a cycle of oral steroid use to calm down the flares. They also can lead to significant systemic adverse effects, hypothalamus-pituitary-adrenal axis suppression, growth retardation, weight gain, obesity, and diabetes, in addition to the skin effects that can be seen with TCS. Oral steroids should be avoided in the treatment of eczema.[28]

Oral immunosuppressants
For severe, recalcitrant eczema immunosuppressant therapy may be helpful in controlling flares. These therapies should be reserved for patients who have not responded to other treatments because they do carry the risk for potentially severe side effects. In this section the authors review 4 of the most commonly prescribed immunosuppressants used in severe eczema. All of these medications are used as off-label treatments.

Cyclosporine

Cyclosporine is a potent T-cell inhibitor and was originally used to prevent rejection in transplant patients. It has been used as off-label in the treatment of refractory eczema with moderate success.

Initial pediatric dosing should be 3 to 6 mg/kg/d and improvement should be seen within 2 to 6 weeks of initiating therapy. Nephrotoxicity and hepatotoxicity should be monitored for with baseline levels and repeat levels every 2 weeks for the first 3 months and then monthly thereafter. Common side effects include elevated blood pressure, headaches, hypertrichosis, and gingival hyperplasia. Therapy can be short-term (3 months) or long-term (12 months).[28]

Azathioprine

Azathioprine is a purine analogue that affects DNA synthesis in rapidly proliferating cells including T cells. It has been used in refractory eczema with modest success. Metabolism of azathioprine involves an enzyme called thiopurine methyltransferase. Low enzyme levels can lead to toxicity and should be evaluated before starting this medication.

Initial pediatric dosing should be 2.5 to 4 mg/kg/d. Common adverse effects include nausea and vomiting and headache. More severe side effects can include hepatotoxicity and leukopenia. It is recommended to check liver function tests, renal function, and complete blood counts before starting treatment. They should be reevaluated twice monthly for the first 2 to 3 months and then monthly after that. This treatment should not be used in conjunction with phototherapy, as there is a risk of skin malignancy with ultraviolet A (UVA) exposure.[28]

Methotrexate

Methotrexate is an antifolate metabolite that can affect T-cell function through disruption of DNA and RNA synthesis. Improvement in symptom scores is generally seen over 10 to 12 weeks. It can be given in oral or injectable form, based on patient preference.

Studies have shown improvement in eczema symptom scores with varying doses of methotrexate, which leads to a wide range of recommended dosing. Initial dosing ranges from 0.2 to 0.7 mg/kg/wk. Severe adverse effects include myelosuppression, hepatotoxicity, and pulmonary fibrosis. Laboratories should be followed with a complete blood count and liver function weekly for the first month. Once stable, laboratories can be checked every 3 months. If patients develop a cough, consider performing a chest radiograph to evaluate for pulmonary fibrosis.[28]

Mycophenolate mofetil

Mycophenolate mofetil (MMF) blocks purine biosynthesis and preferentially affects T and B cells. There have been variable results for the efficacy of MMF. Overall studies show that it can be an option of refractory eczema.

Dosing used in studies has been variable, so the initial dosing can range from 30 to 50 mg/kg/d. Adverse reactions include headaches and GI upset. Rarely it can cause leukopenia. It is recommended to check complete blood counts, renal function, and hepatic function every 2 weeks for the first month and then monthly.[28]

Phototherapy

Another option for patients with refractory eczema is phototherapy. This involves use of UVA, ultraviolet B (UVB), or a combination of both. UVB therapy is the most commonly used and can be narrow or broad band. Unfortunately, because of the dearth of head-to-head trials, there are no guidelines on the most efficacious option.

Phototherapy can be used in conjunction with other therapies except TCIs and azathioprine.

Narrowband UVB is the preferred therapy, as it has lower risk profile. Use of UVA and UVA with UVB contain the most risk.

The major side effects associated with phototherapy include redness and burning at the site of exposure, actinic damage, rashes, and rarely malignancy. Therapy regimens vary depending on the type of UV exposure and can be used both intermittently and chronically.[28]

Phototherapy should be administered by an appropriate facility and the options of phototherapy may be limited by local availability.

Biologics

Biological therapies are novel treatment options that have been emerging for eczema. These therapies have a specific mechanism of action and can target the underlying causes of inflammation while minimizing other side effects.

Dupilumab is an injectable monoclonal antibody that blocks both interleukin-4 (IL-4) and IL-13. Both IL-4 and IL-13 have been implicated in atopic inflammation and believed to be a driving force for eczematous inflammation. IL-4 has been shown in in vitro studies to upregulate other inflammatory cytokines leading to a defective skin barrier, which is the underlying cause of eczema. IL-13 has been show to be overexpressed in both acute and chronic eczematous lesions.[29]

Two trials, SOLO 1 and SOLO 2, were performed to evaluate for the efficacy of dupilumab in comparison to placebo on patients with moderate to severe eczema. Patients were given the medication weekly or every other week. There was a statistically significant improvement in both studies in subjective symptoms, signs of eczema, and quality of life. Both regimens showed similar efficacy as well.[30] Another study looked at the safety profile of dupilumab with concomitant TCI and TCS use. Twice weekly and weekly dosing of dupilumab was compared with placebo. Although they showed that 39% of patients in both treatment arms achieved significant improvement in their eczema, they did note there was a higher incidence of noninfectious conjunctivitis in the dupilumab group.[31] This echoed a similar finding in the SOLO 1 and SOLO 2 trials that also showed a higher incidence of conjunctivitis.

The most common side effect of dupilumab is injection site reaction. It is unclear what the underlying cause of the increased conjunctivitis is in the patients treated with dupilumab, but this phenomenon was only seen in the trials for eczema and was not seen in dupilumab trials for other conditions such as asthma.[30]

At this time, unfortunately, dupilumab is only approved for adult patients with eczema. Pediatric trials are currently underway.

Antihistamines

Pruritus is one of the hallmark signs of eczema and can lead to significant decrease in quality of life for patients with eczema. Although histamine released from mast cells is a known cause of pruritus in atopic disease, it does not seem to be the only or leading cause of pruritus in eczema. Neuropeptides and bradykinin have been identified as inducers of pruritus in eczematous lesions, whereas histamine seems to have only a small effect.[32,33] Antihistamines may not provide significant relief of pruritus but can be useful with sleep disturbance secondary to pruritus. First-generation antihistamines, which have a sedating effect, can provide some relief at night and help decrease scratching, which can worsen symptoms. Use of these antihistamines during the day, however, can be problematic because of sedation.

Table 4
The severity of eczema and the corresponding treatment options

Severity of Eczema	Therapeutic Options
Mild	Good skin care and moisturization
	Mild potency topical steroids for flares
Moderate	Bleach baths
	Moderate potency topical steroids
	Topical calcineurin inhibitors
	Crisaborole
Severe	Wet wraps
	Phototherapy
	Systemic immunosuppresants
	Dupilumab

Management

Eczema is a chronic relapsing disease secondary to an impaired skin barrier. Management requires maintenance therapy to maintain the skin barrier as well as a variety of pharmacologic therapies to help treat flares. For patients with recalcitrant eczema, determining if it is primary eczema versus part of a different disease process is important. Newer biological therapies offer effective results with fewer side effects than systemic oral immunomodulators and steroids. Determining the severity of eczema and underlying triggers will not only help decrease flares but also help determine the best course of treatment (**Table 4**).

REFERENCES

1. Shaw T, Currie G, Koudelka C, et al. Eczema prevalence in the United States: data from the 2003 national survey of children. J Invest Dermatol 2011;131: 67–73.

2. Bieber T. Atopic dermatitis. N Engl J Med 2008;358:1483–94.

3. Maliyar K, Sibbald C, Pope E, et al. Diagnosis and management of atopic dermatitis: a review. Adv Skin Wound Care 2018;(12):538–50.

4. Eichenfield LF, Tom WL, Chamlin SL, et al. Guidelines of care for the management of atopic dermatitis: section 1. Diagnosis and assessment of atopic dermatitis. J Am Acad Dermatol 2014;70(2):338–51.

5. Kunz B, Oranje AP, Labreze L, et al. Clinical validation and guidelines for the SCORAD index: consensus report of the European Task Force on Atopic Dermatitis. Dermatology 1997;195:10–9.

6. Siegfried EC, Hebert AA. Diagnosis of atopic dermatitis: mimics, overlaps, and complications. J Clin Med 2015;4(5):884–917.

7. Eichenfield LF, Tom WL, Berger TG, et al. Guidelines of care for the management of atopic dermatitis: section 2. Management and treatment of atopic dermatitis with topical therapies. J Am Acad Dermatol 2014;71(1):116–32.

8. Draelos ZD. The science behind skin care: moisturizers. J Cosmet Dermatol 2018;17(2):138–44.

9. Chopra R, Vakharia PP, Sacotte R, et al. Efficacy of bleach baths in reducing atopic dermatitis: a systemic review and meta-analysis. Ann Allergy Asthma Immunol 2017;119(5):435–40.

10. Shi VY, Foolad N, Ornelas JN, et al. Comparing the effect of bleach and water baths on skin barrier function in atopic dermatitis: a split-body randomized controlled trial. Br J Dermatol 2016;175(1):212–4.
11. Nicol NH, Boguniewicz M. Wet wrap therapy in moderate to severe atopic dermatitis. Immunol Allergy Clin North Am 2017;37(1):123–39.
12. Janmohamed SR, Oranje AP, Devillers AC, et al. The proactive wet-wrap method with diluted corticosteroids versus emollients in children with atopic dermatitis: a prospective, randomized, double-blind, placebo-controlled trial. J Am Acad Dermatol 2014;70(6):1076–82.
13. Sampson HA. Role of immediate food hypersensitivity in the pathogenesis of atopic dermatitis. J Allergy Clin Immunol 1983;71:473–80.
14. Burks AW, Mallory SB, Williams LW, et al. Atopic dermatitis: clinical relevance of food hypersensitivity reactions. J Pediatr 1988;113:447–51.
15. Robison RG, Singh AM. Controversies in allergy: food testing and dietary avoidance in atopic dermatitis. J Allergy Clin Immunol Pract 2019;7(1):35–9.
16. Chang A, Robison R, Cai M, et al. Natural history of food-triggered atopic dermatitis and development of immediate reactions in children. J Allergy Clin Immunol Pract 2016;4:229–36.e1.
17. Darsow U, Laifaoui J, Kerschenlohr K, et al. The prevalence of positive reactions in the atopy patch test with aeroallergens and food allergens in subjects with atopic eczema: a European multicenter study. Allergy 2004;59:1318–25.
18. Tan BB, Weald D, Strickland I, et al. Double-blind controlled trial of effect of housedust-mite allergen avoidance on atopic dermatitis. Lancet 1996;347:15–8 (Ib).
19. Oosting AJ, de Bruin-Weller MS, Terreehorst I, et al. Effect of mattress encasings on atopic dermatitis outcome measures in a double-blind, placebo-controlled study: the Dutch mite avoidance study. J Allergy Clin Immunol 2002;110:500–6 (Ib).
20. Hostetler SG, Kaffenberger B, Hostetler T, et al. The role of airborne proteins in atopic dermatitis. J Clin Aesthet Dermatol 2010;3(10):22–31.
21. Admani S, Jacob SE. Allergic contact dermatitis in children: review of the past decade. Curr Allergy Asthma Rep 2014;14:421.
22. Milam EC, Jacob SE, Cohen DE. Contact dermatitis in the patient with atopic dermatitis. J Allergy Clin Immunol Pract 2019;7(1):18–26.
23. Long CC, Finlay AY. The finger tip unit- a new practical measure. Clin Exp Dermatol 1991;16(6):444–7.
24. Kusari A, Han AM, Shairer D, et al. Atopic dermatitis: new developments. Dermatol Clin 2019;37(1):11–20.
25. Paller AS, Tom WL, Lebwohl MG, et al. Efficacy and safety of crisaborole ointment, a novel, nonsteroidal phosphodiesterase 4 (PDE4) inhibitor for the topical treatment of atopic dermatitis (AD) in children and adults. J Am Acad Dermatol 2016;75(3):494–503.e6.
26. Totte JE, van der Feltz WT, Hennekam M, et al. Prevalence and odds of Staphylococcus aureus carriage in atopic dermatitis: a systematic review and meta-analysis. Br J Dermatol 2016;175:687–95.
27. Darabi K, Hostetler SG, Bechtel MA, et al. The role of Malassezia in atopic dermatitis affecting the head and neck of adults. J Am Acad Dermatol 2009;60:125–36.
28. Sidbury R, Davis DM, Cohen DE, et al. Guidelines of care for the management of atopic dermatitis: section 3. Management and treatment with phototherapy and systemic agents. J Am Acad Dermatol 2014;71(2):327–49.

29. Brandt E, Sivaprasad U. Th2 cytokines and atopic dermatitis. J Clin Cell Immunol 2011;2(3):110.
30. Simpson EL, Bieber T, Guttman-Yassky E, et al. Two phase 3 trials of dupilumab versus placebo in atopic dermatitis. N Engl J Med 2016;375(24):2335–48, 69.
31. Blauvelt A, de Bruin-Weller M, Gooderham M, et al. Long-term management of moderate-to-severe atopic dermatitis with dupilumab and concomitant topical corticosteroids (LIBERTY AD CHRONOS): a 1-year, randomized, double-blinded, placebo-controlled, phase 3 trial. Lancet 2017;389(10086):2287–303.
32. Buddenkotte J, Steinhoff M. Pathophysiology and therapy of pruritus in allergic and atopic diseases. Allergy 2010;65(7):805–21.
33. Hosogi M, Schmelz M, Miyachi Y, et al. Bradykinin is a potent pruritogen in atopic dermatitis: a switch from pain to itch. Pain 2006;126(1):16–23.

What to Do with an Abnormal Newborn Screen for Severe Combined Immune Deficiency

Hey J. Chong, MD, PhD[a],*, Scott Maurer, MD[a],
Jennifer Heimall, MD[b]

KEYWORDS

- Severe combined immunodeficiency • Newborn screen • SCID screen protocol

KEY POINTS

- Screening for severe combined immunodeficiency identifies infants with naïve T-cell lymphopenia.
- There is state-to-state variability in the assay methodology and reporting of these screens, and institution-to-institution variability in follow-up, so it is helpful for immunologists to understand the protocols in their own state.
- Primary care providers and immunologists need to be prepared to manage these families as a whole, with care and attention to disclosure as well as workup and management.

INTRODUCTION

Definition of Severe Combined Immunodeficiency

Severe combined immunodeficiency (SCID) is the descriptive name for a group of severe inborn errors of immunity characterized by poor T-and B-cell production and/or function resulting in susceptibility to life threatening infections.[1] Without definitive therapy before the age of 1 year, SCID is typically fatal. There are now at least 20 known monogenetic causes of SCID, and genetic testing should be performed early after the clinical diagnosis is made. SCID is a clinical diagnosis; however, the identification of a gene is helpful to guide therapy options including use of alkylator based conditioning

Financial Disclosures: The authors have indicated they have no financial relationships relevant to this article to disclose.
[a] Department of Pediatrics, UPMC Children's Hospital of Pittsburgh, 4401 Penn Avenue, Pittsburgh, PA 15224, USA; [b] Division of Allergy and Immunology, Children's Hospital of Philadelphia, Wood 3301, 3401 Civic Center Boulevard, Philadelphia, PA 19104, USA
* Corresponding author. Department of Pediatrics, Division of Allergy and Immunology, UPMC Children's Hospital of Pittsburgh, 4401 Penn Avenue, Pittsburgh, PA 15224.
E-mail address: hey.chong@chp.edu

Immunol Allergy Clin N Am 39 (2019) 535–546
https://doi.org/10.1016/j.iac.2019.07.007
0889-8561/19/© 2019 Elsevier Inc. All rights reserved.
immunology.theclinics.com

before hematopoietic stem cell transplantation, gene therapy, or, in the case of SCID owing to adenosine deaminase deficiency, enzyme replacement therapy.[2,3]

The Primary Immunodeficiency Treatment Consortium set diagnostic criteria for typical SCID as fewer than 300 T cells/μL and less than 10% of normal phytohemagluttinin proliferative responses, and/or maternal T-cell engraftment.[4] For leaky SCID, patients present with significant impairment of T cells, but unlike typical SCID, have greater than 300 T cells/μL, and no maternal T-cell engraftment.[4] Some of these patients experience a peripheral expansion of oligoclonal T cells, leading to an almost graft-versus-host–like clinical picture with autoreactive T-cell infiltration of skin and gut, alopecia, erythroderma, hepatosplenomegaly, and lymphadenopathy. When this occurs, this clinical presentation is called Omenn syndrome.[3] Leaky SCID occurs as a result of hypomorphic mutations in typical SCID-causing genes, most commonly the recombination activating genes (RAG1 or RAG2) genes.[4,5] Omenn syndrome requires the use of immunosuppression to avoid life-threatening complications from these autoreactive T cells.[6]

SEVERE COMBINED IMMUNODEFICIENCY SCREEN HISTORY

It has been known for the last 20 years that the best outcomes for SCID patients are associated with hematopoietic stem cell transplantation early in life, before the onset of infections. Infants transplanted in the first 3 months of life have been found to have a greater than 95% survival compared with 74% of those transplanted after the neonatal period.[7] These data spurned efforts to advocate for universal screening for SCID, but the lack of a cost-effective and sensitive assay prohibited its addition to the newborn screening panel.[8] In 2005, it was determined that T-cell receptor excision circles (TRECs) could successfully be detected from DNA samples derived from dried blood spot samples on Guthrie cards.[9,10] These cards were already the mechanism of blood collection used throughout the United States to perform a host of screens for varied severe diseases. The TREC screen is a quantitative polymerase chain reaction assay, which measures the byproducts of the T-cell receptor V-D-J rearrangement. Because TRECs can only be detected in naïve T cells recently emigrated from the thymus, low TREC copies in the dried blood spot would indicate naïve T-cell lymphopenia, which is a feature of SCID, among other conditions.[10] The assay is both highly sensitive and specific, with a false-positive rate owing to amplification failure of less than 0.1%.[11] With the validation of this high-throughput DNA based assay, the SCID screen was nominated to the Secretary's Advisory Committee on Heritable Disorders in Newborns and Children in 2007 for addition to the Recommended Universal Screening Panel. Wisconsin was the first state to pilot SCID screening in January 2008, with a second statewide pilot initiated in Massachusetts a year later. A third pilot study in 2009 screened 2000 births at 2 Arizona hospitals in the Navajo reservation, which was selected owing to the high rates of ARTEMIS SCID in this population, to increase the likelihood of detecting true SCID patients during the pilot period. Data collected from these pilots lead to the recommendation of the SCID screen to the Recommended Universal Screening Panel in January 2010, and by fall of 2010, a national pilot SCID study was initiated. In May of 2011, the Secretary's Advisory Committee on Heritable Disorders in Newborns and Children submitted a report on the progress of the 6 states and 1 territory performing newborn screening for SCID.[12] Of the 961,925 newborns screened, 14 cases of SCID had been identified, with an additional 6 patients reported as having an SCID variant. In addition, 40 newborns were identified as non-SCID lymphopenia, with 30% of those being 22q11.2 deletion syndrome, 35% reported as idiopathic T-cell lymphopenia, 5% trisomy 21, and the other 30% as other.

Of importance, no missed cases of SCID were reported.[12] With the success of this pilot, other states started adding the SCID screen to the newborn screening panel, and now as of the end of 2018, all 50 states are screening for SCID, as well as Puerto Rico (**Fig. 1**).

The majority of infants identified through abnormal SCID screens have a non-SCID cause of lymphopenia. In 2014, data from more than 3 million infants screened in 11 programs across the country was reported.[10] This report highlighted that there was variability to the methodology for TREC testing assays and cutoffs used to define lymphopenia on follow-up flow cytometry, despite most programs adhering to the Clinical and Laboratory Standards Institute guidelines available at that time. Of the 1265 patients referred for flow cytometry in this large cohort, 52 were found to have SCID (42 typical SCID, 10 leaky SCID) and 411 were found to have non-SCID lymphopenia. Recognized congenital syndromes associated with lymphopenia were found in 136 of the 411 infants with non-SCID lymphopenia. Of these infants, 78 patients were diagnosed with 22q11.2 deletion syndrome and 21 patients with trisomy 21. One hundred seventeen infants with non-SCID lymphopenia had secondary T-cell lymphopenia from other congenital issues—such as cardiac anomalies or multiple congenital anomalies—or intestinal development defects leading to potential loss of T cells—such as gastroschisis or intestinal atresias. Preterm birth alone was responsible for 29 cases of non-SCID lymphopenia.[13] In California, although only 9% of all newborns screened are in the neonatal intensive care unit, these infants accounted for one-half of the abnormal TREC screens requiring further testing through lymphocyte subset enumeration.[2] The most recent report of SCID screening in California found similar populations of positive SCID screens. Of the more than 3.2 million newborns tested in the state over 7 years, 213 patients were identified with T-cell lymphopenia. Of these patients, 50 were diagnosed with SCID and 72 patients with syndromes or other inborn errors of immunity. They also reported originally 55 with idiopathic lymphopenia, with further follow-up identifying syndromes in 22 of these infants. Of the 33 patients with true idiopathic lymphopenia, 13 resolved or improved over time.[13]

WHAT TO DO WITH AN ABNORMAL SEVERE COMBINED IMMUNODEFICIENCY SCREEN
Understand the T-cell Receptor Excision Circles Assay Implementation in Your State

To most effectively guide patients through the journey of notification of an abnormal SCID newborn screening (NBS), follow-up testing and definitive diagnosis, it is critical that all immunologists understand the SCID screen methodology and algorithm in their own state.

Who Is Being Screened?

It is important to note that having SCID screening added to the state panel does not guarantee that every infant born in the state is screened. For example, in Pennsylvania, the SCID screen is not mandatory in every hospital and birthing center. Unfortunately, there have been previously described 2 cases of classic SCID born to Pennsylvania-based families since the official start of the statewide SCID NBS program. Of these, 2 were born at Pennsylvania hospitals that opted out of screening, and they presented with severe infections later in life. Fortunately, both patients have since been treated with hematopoietic stem cell transplantation, but one has permanent visual impairment owing to cytomegalovirus (CMV) infection. As of this writing, there are still 11 hospitals who do not screen for SCID (personal communication, Pennsylvania

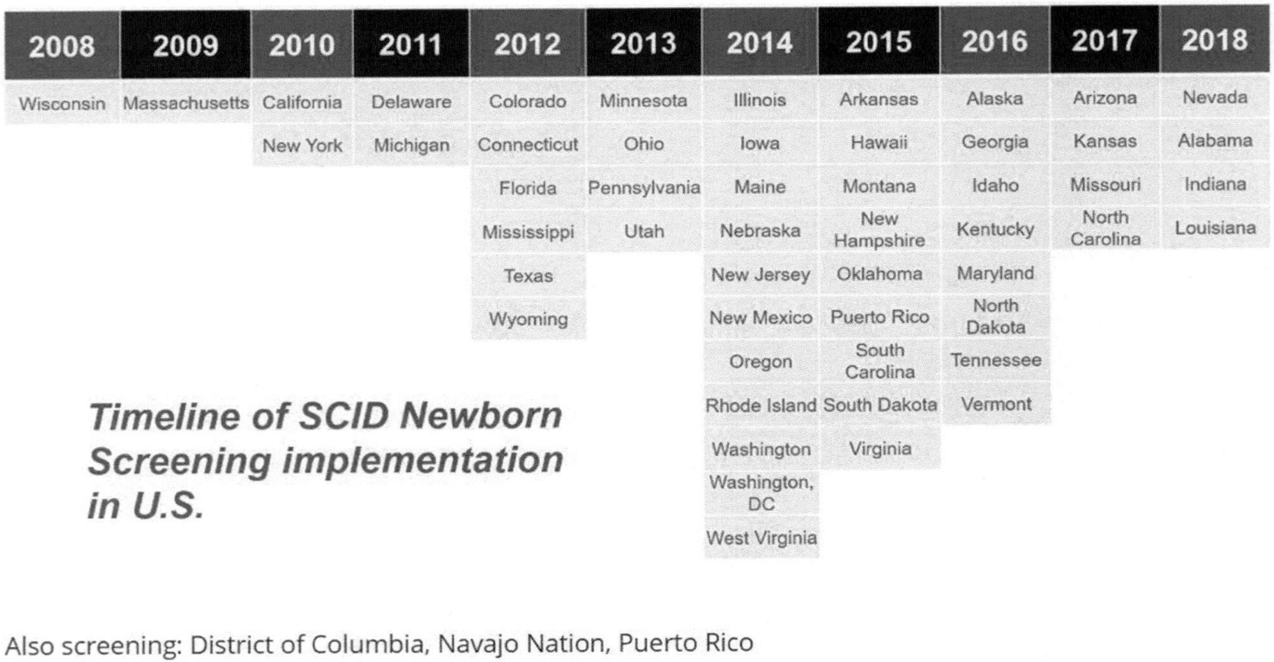

Timeline of SCID Newborn Screening implementation in U.S.

2008	2009	2010	2011	2012	2013	2014	2015	2016	2017	2018
Wisconsin	Massachusetts	California	Delaware	Colorado	Minnesota	Illinois	Arkansas	Alaska	Arizona	Nevada
		New York	Michigan	Connecticut	Ohio	Iowa	Hawaii	Georgia	Kansas	Alabama
				Florida	Pennsylvania	Maine	Montana	Idaho	Missouri	Indiana
				Mississippi	Utah	Nebraska	New Hampshire	Kentucky	North Carolina	Louisiana
				Texas		New Jersey	Oklahoma	Maryland		
				Wyoming		New Mexico	Puerto Rico	North Dakota		
						Oregon	South Carolina	Tennessee		
						Rhode Island	South Dakota	Vermont		
						Washington	Virginia			
						Washington, DC				
						West Virginia				

Also screening: District of Columbia, Navajo Nation, Puerto Rico

Fig. 1. Timeline of SCID newborn screening implementation in the United States. (*From* Immune Deficiency Foundation (IDF). IDF SCID Newborn Screening Campaign. Available at: https://primaryimmune.org/idf-advocacy-center/idf-scid-newborn-screening-campaign. Accessed Feb 15 2019; with permission.)

Department of Health). Data from the Pennsylvania Department of Health from April 1 2017 to March 31 2018 reported that the vast majority of patients born in hospitals and birthing centers now underwent SCID screening, but only 23% of those born to midwives were screened for SCID (**Fig. 2**). Our state also has a population of Amish and Mennonite people who do not routinely have SCID screens available as a part of the newborn screen. We are aware of at least 3 Amish newborns with adenosine deaminase deficiency SCID who were not SCID screened, but were identified through family history. Therefore, it is very important for the immunologist to understand how the SCID screen is implemented in their state, if it is mandated, and if there are populations who are not screened.

Another population to consider are the preterm infants. The screening protocol is not uniform, with some states screening regularly and repeating if less than 37 weeks of gestation, and other states not routinely repeating newborn screens on premature infants.[14] In addition, this population is more likely to have the dried blood spots done from a peripheral line, rather than a heel stick, which can lead to false-positive SCID screens.[14] In Pennsylvania, abnormal SCID screen results in infants less than 37 weeks of gestation are repeated every 4 weeks until 37 weeks of gestation. There is also a very low birth weight algorithm in our state, and newborns born weighing less than 1500 g will receive a repeat specimen at 14 days of age if the first is abnormal.

What Is the Laboratory Methodology for Detection of T-cell Receptor Excision Circles and Quality Control?

There is variability in the TREC assay from state to state, with testing housed in different laboratories, each with their own methodology for testing and quality control.[10] The TREC assay depends on the quality of the dried blood spot on Guthrie cards, and the cellular content and DNA quality can vary as much as 10-fold from the same dried blood spot.[10] It is also known that blood from indwelling catheters can cause an artificial lymphopenia secondary to dilution of the blood sample. In addition, these samples may also contain substances that interfere with quantitative polymerase chain reaction reactions, such as heparin.[15,16] Therefore, amplification of a housekeeping gene from the same sample as the TREC assay confirms DNA quality and presence of cells.[17,18] The reference gene ideally is expressed evenly and constantly, and most SCID screening laboratories use beta-actin or ribonuclease P. Some states such as New York, Texas, Washington, and Massachusetts check an internal reference gene for every sample, whereas other states, such as Wisconsin and Pennsylvania, only amplify the reference gene if the initial TREC assay is abnormal.[14,19]

Severe Combined Immunodeficiency (SCID) Update
May 3, 2018

Newborns Screened for SCID
Most filter papers received by PerkinElmer Genetics between April 1, 2017 and March 31, 2018 were screened for SCID.

	Screened for SCID	Not screened for SCID	Total
Hospitals/Birth Centers	120,664	13,355	134,019
Midwives	990	3,379	4,369
Total	121,654	16,734	138,388

Fig. 2. Newborns screened for SCID in Pennsylvania from April 1, 2017, to March 31, 2018. (*Courtesy of* Pennsylvania Department of Health, Harrisburg, PA.)

Another important variable is the cutoff level used to determine if a SCID screen is abnormal. This TREC and reference gene copy number threshold is different in different states, and where these levels are set will affect the number of false positives. Wisconsin uses a TREC value of 25 to trigger a repeat with beta-actin as a control, and if the beta-actin is normal and TREC count again less than 25, this is reported as abnormal to the primary care provider.[20] California has adjusted their threshold over time and, as of 2017, infants with fewer than 18 TRECS/μL and adequate beta-actin have follow-up lymphocyte subset measurement done as a part of the state NBS program.[2] New York originally used a cutoff value of less than 200 TRECS/μL, but this was lowered to less than 125 TRECs/μL for referral to tertiary centers owing to an unacceptably high false-positive rate with the higher TREC cutoff level.[21]

Pennsylvania has contracted with a commercial laboratory (PerkinElmer) to perform all of the SCID screening in the state. This laboratory uses an initial cutoff of fewer than 40 TREC copies to trigger a repeat of the assay with a beta-actin control. The SCID screen is reported as presumptive positive only if repeat TREC count is less than 25 with a beta-actin result of more than 10,000 copies, but for samples where the beta-actin is also low, these are reported as inconclusive (**Fig. 3**). Communication with the laboratory to understand their methodology and algorithm is very helpful when interpreting results.

WHAT HAPPENS AFTER THERE IS A POSITIVE SEVERE COMBINED IMMUNODEFICIENCY SCREEN?

Once an abnormal TREC count is confirmed and the quality of the sample is assured, there needs to be a clear pathway for patient notification, with defined roles and

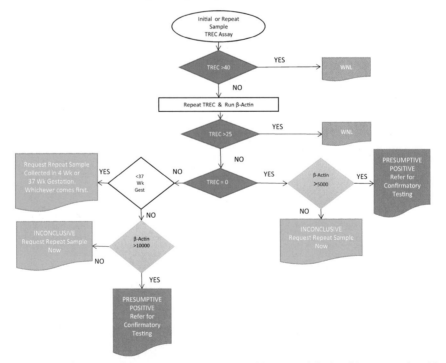

Fig. 3. SCID flowchart for Pennsylvania. WNL. Within normal limits. (*Courtesy of* PerkinElmer Genetics, Pittsburgh, PA.)

responsibilities for the screening laboratory, the state department of health, the primary care provider, and the immunologist. The Pennsylvania Department of Health has contracted with PerkinElmer Genetics for this process, and the genetic counselors notify providers of the results of the SCID screen. The positive report is then also faxed to the designated immunology center.

Without a uniform process, it is not always abundantly clear as to who should be disclosing results to patients, whether it be the department of health, the primary care provider, or the immunologist. In some states such as ours, it is possible for the immunologist to receive the report and contact the family before the primary care provider.

DISCLOSING RESULTS

Depending on the state and the operating protocol for reporting results, immunologists are sometimes the first medical professionals to talk with these families, and these families rely on us to explain the testing results. It is particularly important to be aware of the psychosocial vulnerabilities faced by these families, especially because the results of the screen come at around 2 weeks of life, which coincides with the onset of postpartum depression.[22,23] Delivering serious news to a family can be very stressful and physicians are often not well-trained to handle patient emotions.[24]

Properly conveying SCID screening results requires some degree of preparation and should be treated like other conversations where serious or distressing news is disclosed. In this case, because most of these infants are well-appearing at the time of the SCID screen results, parents are unlikely to expect this conversation, and may experience shock, confusion, and denial. It important to precede the news with a warning, such as, "Your baby's newborn screening results have come back. Is it ok if we sit down and talk about them?" In saying this, the provider indicates to the parent that there is something serious to talk about, but it avoids eliciting an overt emotional response. Further, asking it in the form of a question gives the parent some degree of control of the conversation. At the point of sitting down, the clinician should deliver the news in a concise and clear headline, such as, "One of the tests on your baby's newborn screen shows that he has lower levels of immune cells in his body than normal, and we will have to do further testing to investigate the cause." It is important to avoid the natural tendency to obscure the headline of the conversation with a lot of supporting information, or with providing too much technical information all at once. Hearing this news is likely to cause strong emotions such that continuing at this point would inundate the parent with a tsunami of information that will not be heard or remembered.[25] A better strategy is to pause after giving distressing information and allow the family and patient time to process the information.

When the parent does speak, it is important for the clinician to recognize that the parent is likely in state of emotional distress. Thus, a comment such as, "How could this be possible? He's perfectly healthy!" should be recognized as an emotional response, rather than a request for clarification or more information. A clinician who responds empathetically has the potential to deepen their relationship with the parent and creates supportive collaboration.[26,27] The NURSE method (**Table 1**) is helpful in constructing responses to strong emotions.[28] As opposed to giving more information, simply naming the emotion conveys an understanding of the parent's emotion. "This news is very shocking," can be followed by a statement of understanding such as, "nothing could have prepared you for this." An acknowledgment that the parent's disbelief is valid, or even normal, humanizes the response and shows respect for their

Table 1 The "NURSE" mnemonic		
N	Name	"It sounds like you are angry."
U	Understand	"I cannot imagine what you're going through."
R	Respect	"I see how hard you have been fighting for her."
S	Support	"I'm here for you."
E	Explore	"Tell me more about what you're thinking."

This mnemonic provides guidance for constructing responses to strong emotion in difficult conversations.
Adapted from University of Washington. Medical Oncology Communication Skills Training. Fundamental Communication Skills. Learning Module 1. 2002.

role as a good parent to their newborn. The clinician can also offer a supporting statement, such as, "although this news is scary, I am with you in this, and we will work together to get more answers." Responding in this way gives the parents the opportunity to move from an emotional to a cognitive mode of thinking. At that point, the clinician can ask, "is it ok if we talk about what this test does and does not mean, and how we will get more information?" Doing so gives control of the conversation back to the parent and allows the physician the opportunity to determine where best to start with more detailed information.

Collaboration with supportive care physicians to provide training on disclosing results and providing emotional support to these families can be helpful. In addition, the Immune Deficiency Foundation, a patient advocacy group, has several patient education materials available to help explain the significance of an abnormal SCID NBS test.

EARLY MANAGEMENT AND DIAGNOSTIC TESTING OF THE INFANT WITH A POSITIVE SEVERE COMBINED IMMUNODEFICIENCY SCREEN

There are several excellent published SCID screen protocols, including those from Wisconsin,[29] New York,[30] and California.[23] There is no set universal protocol, with most institutions adapting their own. Nonetheless, despite differences in implementation and methodology, the general goals of the protocol are the same: to prevent infection, identify the cause of the T-cell lymphopenia, and initiate the most effective treatment possible at an optimal time.

Laboratory Assessment

The first step of a positive SCID screen is confirmatory testing via flow cytometry to enumerate T, B, and natural killer cells. In California, this flow cytometry includes enumeration of naïve T cells in addition to the more general CD3, CD4, and CD8 markers for T cells. The testing is done in a central laboratory even before an immunology consultation is initiated, whereas other states rely on the tertiary referral center to do confirmatory testing.[11,20] Wisconsin's approach is to send for a repeat TREC screen at the initial visit, as well as lymphocyte enumeration of CD4, CD8, and naïve T cells, along with CD19 B cells and CD56 natural killer cells. If T-cell lymphopenia is confirmed, chimerism to assess for maternal engraftment, T-cell mitogen responses, and IgG, IgA, and IgM levels are checked to assess B-cell function before the start of immunoglobulin replacement. Genetic testing is sent once the patient is confirmed to have severe T-cell lymphopenia.[29] In California, lymphocyte enumeration is centralized, and no intervention is taken if T cells are greater than 1500, or if more than

200 naïve CD4 T cells are present. If there are fewer than 200 naïve T cells, the patient is admitted for further workup and management. If the T-cell count greater than 200 but less than 1500, these patients are referred to tertiary centers for further evaluation of the T-cell lymphopenia.[23]

At Children's Hospital of Pittsburgh, in addition to flow cytometry to enumerate lymphocyte subsets and naïve T cells, first-pass testing for all positive SCID screens include IgG, IgA, IgM, and IgE as well as lymphocyte mitogen stimulation with conca-valin A, phytohemagluttinin, and pokeweed. Further testing is initiated depending on likelihood of SCID versus other cause for a positive screen. At Children's Hospital of Philadelphia, our initial assessment includes enumeration of CD4, CD8, naïve, and memory T cells, B cells, natural killer, cells and phytohemagluttinin mitogen prolifera-tion. If this testing returns with cell counts and function consistent with SCID or T-cell lymphopenia, additional testing is performed.

Another important part of the diagnostic process is a thorough history and physical examination. A maternal history can reveal factors that influence T-cell numbers, such as immunosuppressive medications or certain conditions that may influence develop-ment of certain syndromes, such as maternal diabetes. For instance, California iden-tified infants with abnormal TREC screens owing to maternal use of azathioprine and fingolimid during pregnancy.[13]

A thorough family history asking about consanguinity, immune deficiencies, sudden infant death syndrome, cancers, and autoimmune disease could help to guide the diagnostic workup. For example, we evaluated an infant with abnormal SCID NBS, who demonstrated T-cell lymphopenia but was later found to have near normal lymphocyte proliferation to mitogens. In this case, a history of early cancers on both sides of the family guided us to send for flow cytometry–based radiosensitivity testing. The flow cytometry assay revealed impairment of DNA repair, leading to targeted sequencing of the ATM gene and confirmation of ataxia telangiectasia at less than 2 months of age.[31]

A thorough physical examination could reveal features consistent with trisomy 21 or 22q11.2 deletion syndrome. A thorough physical examination could also identify the causes of secondary lymphopenia, through loss, cardiac, or gastrointestinal anoma-lies.[11] In addition, a good history and physical examination should ascertain if the in-fant exhibits any signs or symptoms of illness, which should lead to prompt hospitalization and initiation of further workup and treatment.

ANTICIPATORY GUIDANCE

While the workup is ongoing, supportive care and anticipatory guidance should be provided to families with a focus on infection prevention. Patients should avoid day care, limit contact with younger children, and practice good hand hygiene and other avoidance measures while the confirmatory testing is pending.[20] In addition, during the workup, patients and close household members should avoid live vaccines, and family members should be up to date on killed vaccines, with an emphasis on influenza and diphtheria.

Breastfeeding guidance while evaluation of the patient with an abnormal SCID NBS is ongoing is a controversial topic owing to risk of CMV transmission from a seropos-itive mother to the infant through breastfeeding.[32] This risk is well-known and can be fatal to an infant with SCID. This risk, however, should be balanced with the fact that breastfeeding has benefit to both the mother and the baby, with some studies sug-gesting that breastfeeding can help to prevent postpartum depression.[22] In addition, the majority of infants with positive SCID screens do not actually have SCID, but have

T-cell lymphopenia from other causes, with the most common being congenital syndromes.[33] Data are needed to understand the impact of withholding, sometimes for several weeks while the workup is ongoing. Ideally, the mother can continue to pump and store breast milk until her CMV status is confirmed. Another option is to consider banked breastmilk. Some of these centers use the Holder method of pasteurization, which prevents the transmission of disease including CMV, while maintaining its immunologic bioactivity.[34] This option, if available through a local breastmilk bank, provides an option to mothers to pasteurize her own supply to safely provide to the infant, without needing to wait for testing results.

SUMMARY

The SCID screen saves lives by identifying these infants before the onset of illness and has been proven successful over the last decade to be able to detect SCID patients. In fact, based on TREC-based NBS for SCID, we now know that this disease, although rare, is much more common than prior published estimates. All 50 states are screening, but there is no universal protocol for testing, critical value cutoffs, or follow-up evaluation. Therefore, variability exists state to state.

Knowing what to do with an abnormal SCID screen requires the immunologist to be intimately familiar with the methodology and reporting algorithm in their state. Immunologists would benefit from training in giving serious news to patients, which can help establish a trusting relationship with the family. Immunologists should also be critically involved with the development of protocols at their own institution for the evaluation and initial management of patients with abnormal TREC-based SCID NBS, with input from infectious disease as well as bone marrow transplant specialists as needed.

FUTURE CONSIDERATIONS/SUMMARY

SCID screening is now in all 50 states as well as in several countries, with differences in testing methodology, reporting protocols, and the assessment of these infants once the screen is reported to be abnormal. More data are needed to create universal guidelines for implementation and screening to determine best practices.

REFERENCES

1. Buckley RH. Advances in the understanding and treatment of human severe combined immunodeficiency. Immunol Res 2000;22(2–3):237–51.
2. Puck JM. Newborn screening for severe combined immunodeficiency and T-cell lymphopenia. Immunol Rev 2019;287(1):241–52.
3. Villa A, Notarangelo LD, Roifman CM. Omenn syndrome: inflammation in leaky severe combined immunodeficiency. J Allergy Clin Immunol 2008;122(6):1082–6.
4. Chinn IK, Shearer WT. Severe combined immunodeficiency disorders. Immunol Allergy Clin North Am 2015;35(4):671–94.
5. Dvorak CC, Haddad E, Buckley RH, et al. The genetic landscape of severe combined immunodeficiency in the United States and Canada in the current era (2010-2018). J Allergy Clin Immunol 2019;143(1):405–7.
6. Mazzolari E, Moshous D, Forino C, et al. Hematopoietic stem cell transplantation in Omenn syndrome: a single-center experience. Bone Marrow Transplant 2005;36(2):107–14.
7. Myers LA, Patel DD, Puck JM, et al. Hematopoietic stem cell transplantation for severe combined immunodeficiency in the neonatal period leads to superior thymic output and improved survival. Blood 2002;99(3):872–8.

8. Buckley RH. The long quest for neonatal screening for severe combined immuno-deficiency. J Allergy Clin Immunol 2012;129(3):597–604 [quiz: 605–6].

9. Guthrie R, Susi A. A simple phenylalanine method for detecting phenylketonuria in large populations of newborn infants. Pediatrics 1963;32:338–43.

10. Chan K, Puck JM. Development of population-based newborn screening for se-vere combined immunodeficiency. J Allergy Clin Immunol 2005;115(2):391–8.

11. Puck JM, Routes J, Filipovich AH, et al. Expert commentary: practical issues in newborn screening for severe combined immune deficiency (SCID). J Clin Immu-nol 2012;32(1):36–8.

12. Available at: www.hrsa.gov/sites/default/files/hrsa/advisory-committees/heritable-disorders/reports-recommendations/reports/newborn-screening-scid-report.pdf.

13. Amatuni GS, Currier RJ, Church JA, et al. Newborn screening for severe com-bined immunodeficiency and T-cell lymphopenia in California, 2010-2017. Pediat-rics 2019;143(2) [pii:e20182300].

14. Routes J, Verbsky J. Newborn screening for severe combined immunodeficiency. Curr Allergy Asthma Rep 2018;18(6):34.

15. Holodniy M, Kim S, Katzenstein D, et al. Inhibition of human immunodeficiency virus gene amplification by heparin. J Clin Microbiol 1991;29(4):676–9.

16. Chase NM, Verbsky JW, Routes JM. Newborn screening for SCID: three years of experience. Ann N Y Acad Sci 2011;1238:99–105.

17. Radonic A, Thulke S, Mackay IM, et al. Guideline to reference gene selection for quantitative real-time PCR. Biochem Biophys Res Commun 2004;313(4):856–62.

18. Gerstel-Thompson JL, Wilkey JF, Baptiste JC, et al. High-throughput multiplexed T-cell-receptor excision circle quantitative PCR assay with internal controls for detection of severe combined immunodeficiency in population-based newborn screening. Clin Chem 2010;56(9):1466–74.

19. Ding Y, Thompson JD, Kobrynski L, et al. Cost-effectiveness/cost-benefit analysis of newborn screening for severe combined immune deficiency in Washington State. J Pediatr 2016;172:127–35.

20. Verbsky J, Thakar M, Routes J. The Wisconsin approach to newborn screening for severe combined immunodeficiency. J Allergy Clin Immunol 2012;129(3): 622–7.

21. Albin-Leeds S, Ochoa J, Mehta H, et al. Idiopathic T cell lymphopenia identified in New York State newborn screening. Clin Immunol 2017;183:36–40.

22. Stewart DE, Vigod S. Postpartum depression. N Engl J Med 2016;375(22): 2177–86.

23. Dorsey MJ, Dvorak CC, Cowan MJ, et al. Treatment of infants identified as having severe combined immunodeficiency by means of newborn screening. J Allergy Clin Immunol 2017;139(3):733–42.

24. Baile WF, Buckman R, Lenzi R, et al. SPIKES-A six-step protocol for delivering bad news: application to the patient with cancer. Oncologist 2000;5(4):302–11.

25. Jedlicka-Kohler I, Gotz M, Eichler I. Parents' recollection of the initial communica-tion of the diagnosis of cystic fibrosis. Pediatrics 1996;97(2):204–9.

26. Mack JW, Hilden JM, Watterson J, et al. Parent and physician perspectives on quality of care at the end of life in children with cancer. J Clin Oncol 2005; 23(36):9155–61.

27. Hsiao JL, Evan EE, Zeltzer LK. Parent and child perspectives on physician communication in pediatric palliative care. Palliat Support Care 2007;5(4): 355–65.

28. Medical Oncology Communication Skills Training. Fundamental communication skills, learning module, 1, 2002. Available at: http://depts.washington.edu/oncotalk/learn/modules/Modules_01.pdf. 2019.
29. Thakar MS, Hintermeyer MK, Gries MG, et al. A practical approach to newborn screening for severe combined immunodeficiency using the T cell receptor excision circle assay. Front Immunol 2017;8:1470.
30. Vogel BH, Bonagura V, Weinberg GA, et al. Newborn screening for SCID in New York State: experience from the first two years. J Clin Immunol 2014;34(3): 289–303.
31. Cousin MA, Smith MJ, Sigafoos AN, et al. Utility of DNA, RNA, protein, and functional approaches to solve cryptic immunodeficiencies. J Clin Immunol 2018; 38(3):307–19.
32. Hamprecht K, Maschmann J, Vochem M, et al. Epidemiology of transmission of cytomegalovirus from mother to preterm infant by breastfeeding. Lancet 2001; 357(9255):513–8.
33. Kwan A, Abraham RS, Currier R, et al. Newborn screening for severe combined immunodeficiency in 11 screening programs in the United States. JAMA 2014; 312(7):729–38.
34. Lima HK, Wagner-Gillespie M, Perrin MT, et al. Bacteria and bioactivity in holder pasteurized and shelf-stable human milk products. Curr Dev Nutr 2017;1(8): e001438.

Vocal Cord Dysfunction
The Spectrum Across the Ages

Andrej A. Petrov, MD[a],*

KEYWORDS

- Vocal cord dysfunction • Laryngeal hypersensitivity • Asthma mimicker
- Exercise-induced laryngeal obstruction

KEY POINTS

- Vocal cord dysfunction (VCD) is characterized by laryngeal hyperresponsiveness and shares clinical features with chronic refractory cough, muscle tension dysphonia, and globus pharyngeus.
- VCD is one of the key conditions in the differential diagnosis of asthma and exertional dyspnea in children and adults.
- It is frequently misdiagnosed as asthma and/or exercise-induced bronchoconstriction, leading to redundant testing, emergency department visits, and unnecessary medication use.
- Timely VCD diagnosis and treatment improve patient outcomes. The multidisciplinary approach is needed for patients with significant medical and psychological comorbidities.

INTRODUCTION

The term vocal cord dysfunction (VCD) was first coined in 1983 by Christopher and colleagues,[1] who described 5 patients with VCD misdiagnosed with asthma. However, the clinical entity of functional laryngeal obstruction, initially reported in the mid–nineteenth century, has been renamed with various diagnoses, including hysterical croup, Munchausen stridor, pseudoasthma, factitious asthma, and psychogenic stridor.[2] While the VCD terminology has been adopted by allergy and pulmonary specialists, otolaryngologists have used paradoxic vocal fold motion (PVFM) to describe this condition. Most recently, inducible laryngeal obstruction (ILO) has been suggested as a term to describe the location of upper airway obstruction more accurately, because functional obstruction can occur in the glottic and supraglottic areas of the

Disclosure: The author has nothing to disclose.
[a] Section of Allergy, Division of Pulmonary, Allergy and Critical Care Medicine, University of Pittsburgh Medical Center, Pittsburgh, PA, USA
* Division of Pulmonary, Allergy and Critical Care Medicine, Department of Medicine, University of Pittsburgh Medical Center, 3459 5th Avenue, NW 628 MUH, Pittsburgh, PA 15213.
E-mail address: petrovaa@upmc.edu

larynx.[3] However, it seems that VCD, PVFM, and ILO will continue to be used interchangeably in the future.[4]

The exact prevalence of VCD in the general population is unknown and has been estimated in 1 study at 4% to 6% with the use of a postal questionnaire survey.[5] There is a 2:1 to 3:1 female predominance and two-thirds are adults and one-third children.[6,7] Exercise-induced VCD (EIVCD) occurs more frequently in adolescents and young adults, with an estimated prevalence of 5.7% to 7.6%.[8,9] Brugman's[7] review of VCD literature from 1967 to 2003 reported that the median age was 34.5 years in adults and 14 years in children. Recent pediatric studies found that 75% of children with VCD were older than 13 years,[10,11] and recent adult studies reported that the average age of patients with VCD referred to the specialty clinics was between 47 and 50 years.[12,13]

PATHOPHYSIOLOGY

For the purpose of this article, VCD is divided into 4 subtypes based on their unique and interdependent aspects of pathophysiology. The subtypes are somatic (psychogenic) VCD, spontaneous VCD, irritant VCD, and exercise-induced laryngeal obstruction (EILO). Although the primary mechanisms of abnormal vocal cord motion remain unknown, all VCD subtypes show exaggerated laryngeal constriction during respiration, when visualized by laryngoscopy.[2]

Psychological or somatoform disorders were suspected as the cause of VCD since the condition was discovered.[14] Subsequent studies have identified that VCD is more common in female children and adults with psychological disorders. It is also frequently associated with social and emotional stressors.[15–17] The prevalence of somatic VCD is lower in children compared with adults, likely because in children the EILO subtype is more common and less frequently associated with psychiatric disease. Furthermore, it seems that other psychological mechanisms, such as type A personality and perfectionism personality traits, could be partly responsible for EILO.[18,19] Recent neuroimaging studies of brain activation showed the link between the limbic system and the larynx in patients with primary muscle tension dysphonia.[20,21] It is highly likely that similar mechanisms play a role in somatic VCD.

Many patients with VCD develop symptoms spontaneously or after exposure to a variety of inhalational triggers. Initially described as the irritable larynx syndrome, laryngeal hypersensitivity paradigm could improve the mechanistic understanding of spontaneous VCD.[22,23] Within this framework of laryngeal dysfunction, affected peripheral and central sensory and motor neural pathways show a decreased reactivity threshold to external stimuli coupled with a heightened protective response. The physiologic response of laryngeal closure to prevent aspiration is exaggerated and occurs even with exposure to innocuous triggers. The origin of laryngeal hypersensitivity remains unknown, although it is speculated that it could be caused by viral neuropathy following an upper respiratory tract infection, or neural plasticity/autonomic imbalance induced by repeated noxious and injurious stimuli.[22,24] Laryngeal functions such as vocalization, cough sensitivity, swallowing function, and vocal cord closure are abnormal across the spectrum of laryngeal hypersensitivity syndrome. The clinical manifestations of laryngeal hypersensitivity include chronic refractory cough, muscle tension dysphonia (MTD), globus pharyngeus, and VCD[23] (**Fig. 1**). The study by Vertigan and colleagues[25] examined the presence of VCD with flexible laryngoscopy in adult patients with chronic cough and MTD. Abnormal vocal cord adduction was present in 36% of patients with MTD during phonation. In patients with chronic cough, the abnormal vocal adduction was seen in 47% of patients at rest and 67% after odor

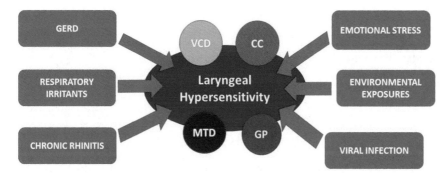

Fig. 1. Various factors that can exacerbate laryngeal hypersensitivity and cause clinical manifestations of VCD, MTD, chronic cough (CC), and globus pharyngeus (GP). GERD, gastroesophageal reflux disease.

challenge. Moreover, the patients with VCD had similar or worse cough testing scores compared with patients with chronic refractory cough.

VCD has been associated with medical comorbidities that may irritate the larynx and contribute to laryngeal hypersensitivity. Two comorbidities frequently implicated are chronic rhinitis and gastroesophageal reflux disease (GERD). The reported prevalence of GERD and chronic rhinitis in pediatric and adult patients with VCD ranges from 14% to 92% and 15% to 75%, respectively.[2,10,12,22,26,27] One study evaluated the presence of sinus disease in VCD and found that there was no significant sinusitis as shown by sinus computed tomography (CT).[28] The frequent finding of vocal cord edema in patients with VCD has been attributed to laryngopharyngeal reflux.[29,30] However, the mechanisms of laryngeal sensitivity in GERD and chronic rhinitis remain to be further elucidated.

Irritant-induced VCD is defined as a subtype of VCD in which a triggering event has been identified as the cause of patient's symptoms.[31] The patients usually report a single significant inhalational exposure to a respiratory irritant, frequently in the occupational setting, followed by new-onset VCD symptoms within 24 hours. The symptoms may recur on exposure to the same irritant or other respiratory irritants. The mechanism remains unknown, although it is postulated that neural plasticity or inflammatory response can develop from epithelial and/or neural injury after workplace exposure to airborne respiratory irritants.[32] The diagnosis is confirmed with an inhalational challenge to an offending chemical and concomitant laryngoscopic visualization of vocal cord adduction.

EILO is defined as an inappropriate transient narrowing of the larynx during exercise resulting in breathing problems. EILO has been reported mostly in adolescents or young adults, which is likely caused by high-intensity exercise more commonly seen in this population. It occurs more often in girls, which could be related to smaller larynx, especially after puberty, compared with boys.[33] The laryngeal obstruction can occur either at the glottic (the true vocal cords) or supraglottic level (the false vocal cords, arytenoid region, and epiglottis), or both.[34] It is suggested that a smaller larynx, with pliable laryngeal cartilage and weaker laryngeal muscles and ligaments, may collapse when exposed to high-volume flow of air during vigorous exercise.[33] Environmental factors such as cold air may play a role because EILO is more frequently seen in outdoor sports.[35] Psychological factors might contribute to the symptoms of EILO, especially in those patients with competitive personality characteristics. However, the association with psychiatric disease is tenuous. For example, the patients who underwent surgical correction of severe supraglottic EILO had significant and lasting improvement of their symptoms.[36]

CLINICAL FEATURES

The clinical presentation may vary between specialties and there is frequently a referral bias present in VCD studies[6,7,10,12,37,38] (**Table 1**). While in adults the symptoms occur more commonly at rest, most children have symptoms with exercise only. For example, resting VCD was seen in 85% of adults and 25% of children, whereas the remainder had EILO.[10,38] Dyspnea is the most common presenting symptom, followed by cough. Dysphonia and difficulty swallowing are complaints more commonly reported to otolaryngologists, whereas wheezing and chest tightness are seen mostly by allergy/immunology and pulmonary medicine specialists. Severe stridor can occur during a severe VCD attack and lead to endotracheal intubation for presumed respiratory failure.[39] This outcome happens mostly in those patients who have not been yet diagnosed with VCD.

Patients with EILO typically develop symptoms during exercise that resolve within several minutes after cessation of exercise. The most common symptom is dyspnea, seen in more than 95% of patients, followed by stridor/hoarseness in 54% of patients.[33] The symptoms progress through several stages, starting with deep inspiratory breathing, followed by dyspnea, and ending with stridor at the peak of exercise.[34] In most patients, the highest obstruction occurs at peak work capacity. Moreover, many patients experience expiratory or biphasic stridor.[40] However, laryngoscopic examination can also show an open glottis in the presence of stridor or shortness of breath induced by an exercise challenge test.[41,42]

DIAGNOSIS

The criteria for diagnosis of VCD combine laryngeal and respiratory symptoms with laryngoscopic visualization of inappropriate vocal cord adduction.[2,3] Pathognomonic findings include inspiratory vocal cord adduction of the anterior two-thirds with a posterior diamond-shaped chink (**Fig. 2**). In the absence of complete glottic obstruction, partial (>50%) inspiratory and/or expiratory vocal cord adduction is considered diagnostic for VCD. Because of the episodic nature of VCD, the examination is frequently normal. According to one review of VCD literature, inspiratory vocal cord adduction was seen in 32% and expiratory adduction in 9% of 978 pediatric and adult patients.[1]

Table 1	
Vocal cord dysfunction symptom profile	
Symptom	**Patients (%)**
Dyspnea	75–98
Cough	40–80
Wheezing	50–80
Chest tightness	15–75
Chest pain	12–22
Throat tightness	15–65
Dysphonia	25–60
Stridor	10–50
Difficulty swallowing	30

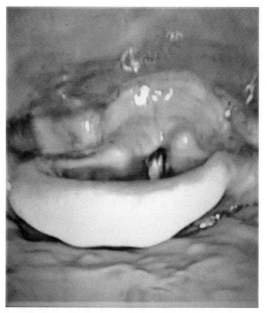

Fig. 2. Pathognomonic finding in VCD: inspiratory vocal cord adduction of the anterior two-thirds with a posterior diamond-shaped chink.

Newman and colleagues[39] reported that laryngoscopy was diagnostic in 60% of asymptomatic adult patients, with 19% showing inspiratory closure, 11% expiratory closure, and 31% showing both inspiratory and expiratory closure of the vocal cords. Maturo and colleagues[10] found that most pediatric patients with resting VCD had a confirmatory laryngoscopic examination for VCD. If laryngoscopy is normal, a provocative challenge with an odor or irritant should be considered to induce abnormal adduction of the vocal cords (**Fig. 3**).

Exercise is an important trigger in VCD. In patients with exercise-induced symptoms only, resting laryngoscopy is usually normal. EILO can be diagnosed with

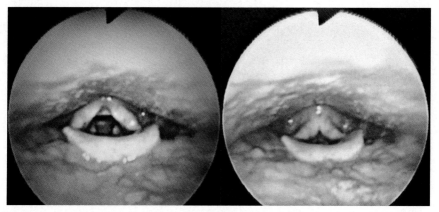

Fig. 3. Vocal cords before (*left*) and after (*right*) a provocative odor challenge. Note complete closure of the vocal cords after exposure to an irritant odor.

postexercise laryngoscopy and/or continuous laryngoscopy with exercise (CLO). The exercise challenge studies are usually performed on the bicycle, treadmill, or during specific sport activities. CLO is considered to be the most sensitive diagnostic method because of its ability to detect short-lived abnormal vocal cord motion in real time.[40] While the reported sensitivity of postexercise laryngoscopy is 50% to 89%,[10,38] CLO can detect EILO in about 85% of patients.[34] The location of obstruction in EILO can be glottic, supraglottic, or both. Whereas Chiang and colleagues[38] reported that laryngeal obstruction was mostly glottic, Røksund and colleagues[34] found that obstruction started in the supraglottic area with secondary involvement of the glottis. Although the symptom of dyspnea was seen with supraglottic obstruction, the stridor developed only if there was adduction of vocal cords.[34] In an adult study, laryngeal closure with exercise was present in 47% of severe asthmatics in all phases of respiration with expiratory closure occurring at the glottic level and inspiratory closure developing mostly at the supraglottic level.[43] The significance and mechanism of expiratory vocal cord closing in asthma seen by either laryngoscopy or dynamic neck CT remain unclear and may not represent a pathologic finding.[44,45]

Vocal Cord Dysfunction and Asthma

Ever since Christopher and colleagues[1] reported a small case series of patients with VCD that was mistaken for asthma, VCD has become preeminent in the differential diagnosis of asthma. VCD can occur in isolation, it can mimic asthma, or it can coexist with asthma. In our study of 132 adult patients with VCD, 42% were misdiagnosed as having asthma for an average of 9 years and 33% had coexistent VCD and asthma.[12] Subjects with VCD misdiagnosed with asthma presented more frequently with shortness of breath, chest tightness, wheezing, and exercise as a trigger compared with those with VCD alone. In addition, this group had higher health care use (HCU), specifically emergency department visits and chest CT imaging studies, and were prescribed more oral steroid courses and inhalers compared with patients with VCD that did not mimic asthma.[46] Newman and colleagues[39] also reported high HCU in their adult VCD cohort and a delay in VCD diagnosis of 4.8 years. Maturo and colleagues[10] published that 44% of children with VCD were labeled erroneously with asthma.

Spirometry can be used to assess airflow through the upper airway. The findings concerning for VCD include flattened or truncated inspiratory flow-volume loops and an abnormal ratio of forced flow at 50% of expiration to forced flow at 50% of inspiration.[6] The frequency of inspiratory flow-volume loop flattening in VCD ranges from 23% to 46%.[1,47] Although it was reported that inspiratory flow-volume loops could be abnormal in patients with VCD during an acute symptomatic phase, other studies found that spirometric findings were unreliable in identifying patients with VCD.[48,49]

As spirometry can be normal in patients with VCD and asthma, it may be necessary to perform bronchoprovocation testing to confirm the correct diagnosis. The most common bronchoprovocation test used is methacholine challenge test, although other agents have been used as well. Methacholine inhalation can cause vocal cord adduction leading to a decrease in lung function. Therefore, whereas a negative methacholine challenge test rules out the diagnosis of asthma, a positive methacholine challenge test can be seen both in VCD and asthma. Laryngoscopy or flow-volume loop interpretation may need to be performed at the time of decline in lung function to evaluate the presence of upper airway obstruction.[47] In addition, it has been the author's experience that a normal exhaled nitric oxide level in the setting of normal spirometry may also help in the process of excluding an asthma diagnosis.

EILO can be misdiagnosed as exercise-induced bronchoconstriction (EIB). While EIB symptoms start after exercise and can last up to 60 minutes, EILO symptoms occur during exercise and resolve promptly on the cessation of exercise. However, a detailed medical history and the presence of inspiratory symptoms were not helpful in distinguishing EILO versus EIB as reported in 2 studies.[10,43] The erroneous diagnosis of EIB was found in 44% to 66% of pediatric patients with EILO/EIVCD.[9–11,35] Importantly, EILO and EIB can coexist in 4% to 12% of patients and bronchial hyperresponsiveness was present in 4% to 26% of subjects with EILO.[9,50] Therefore, clinicians should consider testing for EILO in select patients with EIB who fail to respond to appropriate treatment or in those patients with symptoms suggestive of upper airway obstruction.

VCD is an episodic disease that represents a diagnostic challenge even for those practitioners who are skillful in performing laryngoscopy. For this reason, various questionnaires have been developed to assess the full spectrum of disorders and symptoms that might involve the larynx.[51] Our group has developed the Pittsburgh Vocal Cord Dysfunction Index questionnaire, which has high sensitivity (83%) and specificity (95%) in distinguishing asthma from VCD.[52] (**Fig. 4**) Although laryngoscopy is the gold standard for diagnosing VCD, the implementation of the Pittsburgh VCD Index may facilitate distinguishing VCD from asthma (**Fig. 5**).

Differential Diagnosis

Although most cases of VCD are in one of the 4 groups discussed previously, VCD is infrequently associated with neurologic disease, dysautonomia, Arnold-Chiari syndrome, and mechanical trauma caused by extubation. Laryngomalacia is the most common cause of stridor in neonates and infants. Vocal cord paresis and paralysis should be ruled out during the laryngoscopic examination.[6] Persistent flattening of the inspiratory and expiratory flow-volume loops suggests a fixed cause of upper airway obstruction and requires further evaluation. In one study of adolescents, patients with stridor and normal vocal cord examination were diagnosed with vascular compression, tracheomalacia, and subglottic stenosis.[10] Forrest and colleagues[29] reported that non-VCD diagnoses were seen in 30% of adult patients referred to their

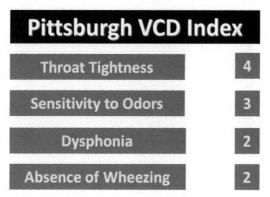

Fig. 4. Pittsburgh VCD Index (positive if score ≥4 points during respiratory symptoms). (*Modified from* Traister RS, Fajt ML, Landsittel D, et al. A novel scoring system to distinguish vocal cord dysfunction from asthma. J Allergy Clin Immunol Pract 2014;2(1):67; with permission.)

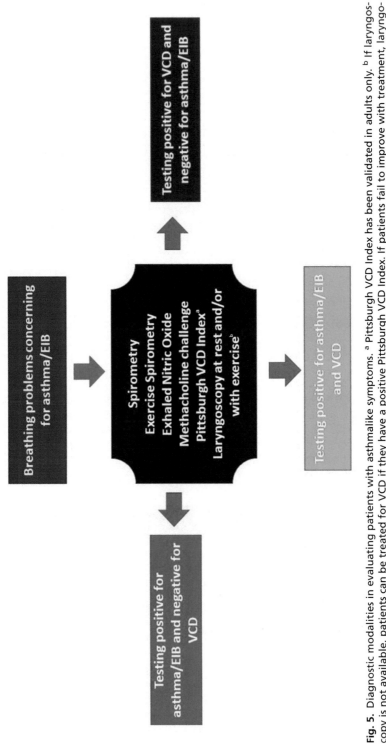

Fig. 5. Diagnostic modalities in evaluating patients with asthmalike symptoms. [a] Pittsburgh VCD Index has been validated in adults only. [b] If laryngoscopy is not available, patients can be treated for VCD if they have a positive Pittsburgh VCD Index. If patients fail to improve with treatment, laryngoscopic examination should be performed to exclude other causes of upper airway obstruction.

center for VCD evaluation. Dysfunctional breathing should also be in the differential diagnosis of VCD, because there is a significant overlap in symptoms between these two conditions.[53] VCD can mimic allergic reactions presenting with upper airway symptoms.[54] VCD symptoms have been described in patients experiencing factitious allergic reactions during drug desensitization or allergen immunotherapy treatments.[55–57] In addition, VCD can coexist with other pulmonary conditions besides asthma. If patients remain symptomatic despite ruling out asthma diagnosis and receiving treatment of VCD, other diagnoses should be investigated.[58]

THERAPY

The cornerstone of VCD therapy consists of a multipronged approach that includes speech and behavioral therapy, treatment of medical comorbidities, and psychological treatment (**Fig. 6**). While most patients require speech and behavioral therapy, targeted additional treatments should be offered if indicated. Most recommendations are based on limited-quality studies and clinical experience, because there is a paucity of randomized controlled studies.[59]

Treatment of acute attacks of VCD starts with reassurance. For many patients, the fear of the unknown and lack of understanding as to why they are experiencing breathing problems contribute to their symptoms and anxiety. The breathing exercises, such as pursed-lip or diaphragmatic breathing, should be attempted to relieve glottic obstruction.[60] If these measures fail, anxiolytics can be used in patients with severe anxiety. Other treatment modalities reported anecdotally to be helpful include 80% helium/20% oxygen mixture (Heliox), continuous positive airway pressure (CPAP), and topical nebulized lidocaine. While CPAP and Heliox may decrease respiratory effort by establishing a favorable pressure gradient for inhalation or decreasing airflow

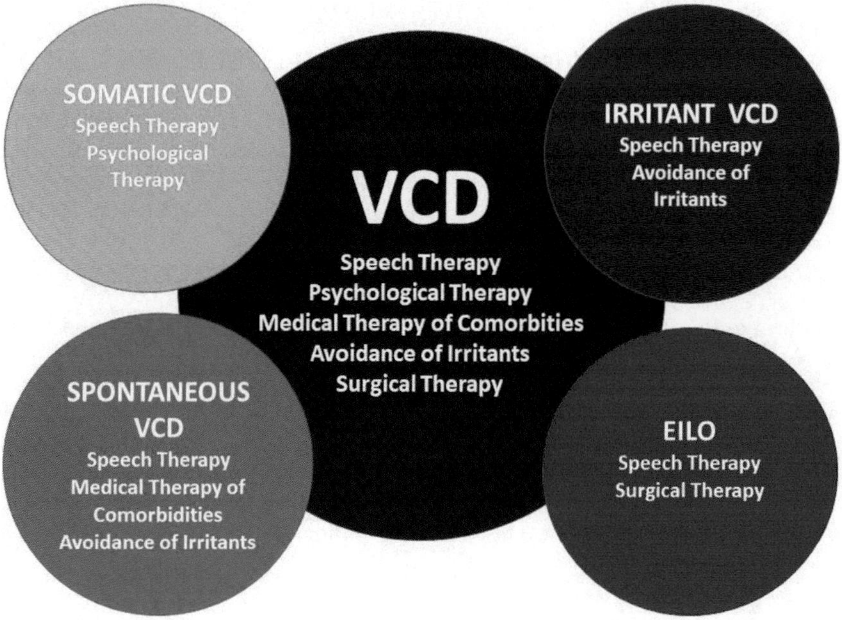

SOMATIC VCD
Speech Therapy
Psychological
Therapy

IRRITANT VCD
Speech Therapy
Avoidance of
Irritants

VCD
Speech Therapy
Psychological Therapy
Medical Therapy of Comorbities
Avoidance of Irritants
Surgical Therapy

SPONTANEOUS VCD
Speech Therapy
Medical Therapy of
Comorbidities
Avoidance of Irritants

EILO
Speech Therapy
Surgical Therapy

Fig. 6. Patients with VCD can be treated with 1 or more treatment modalities based on their clinical presentation.

turbulence in the airway, nebulized lidocaine anesthetizes the upper airway and decreases laryngeal constriction.[47,61] Some patients with VCD, especially those who are unaware of their diagnosis, experience severe respiratory distress requiring intubation. Unlike patients with status asthmaticus, once connected to the mechanical ventilator, they are easy to ventilate.

Chronic therapy for VCD also begins with reassurance. The patients with a history of extensive testing and previous ineffective treatments frequently have a cathartic psychological experience after learning about their VCD diagnosis. Education about VCD, biofeedback, and speech and behavioral therapy represent the first steps in VCD treatment.[60] The reported success rate of speech and behavioral therapy is 68% to 95%, although the number of recommended sessions has not been determined.[10,59,60,62,63] A multidisciplinary approach seems to be most effective in managing patients with VCD, especially in those patients with concomitant asthma or psychological disease.[10,64] One prospective observational study of coexistent asthma and VCD showed decreased inhaler use and improved symptoms with treatment of VCD.[65] Another group reported successful use of inhaled ipratropium for treatment of EIVCD.[63] While there is no uniform approach for testing or treatment, psychological interventions are recommended in children and adults with the somatic component of VCD.[66] Importantly, clinicians should not make an a priori diagnosis of somatic VCD because patients can develop psychiatric disease independent of VCD or because of VCD. In a subset of patients with supraglottic EILO, surgical resection may induce lasting benefit. In a study of adolescents, laser supraglottoplasty was superior to conservative therapy in improving exercise tolerance and decreasing symptoms at 2-year to 5-year follow-up. Although there were no postsurgical complications, the investigators recommended performing this procedure only in highly active athletes with severe supraglottic obstruction.[36] For patients with severe VCD refractory to treatment, botulinum toxin injections have been used. However, tracheostomy procedures have also been reported in the most severe cases.[47]

There are no randomized controlled studies analyzing the association between GERD, chronic rhinitis, and VCD. Two small case series of GERD associated with VCD in infants found that medical treatment of GERD likely had no effect on stridor, and VCD symptoms improved spontaneously with time.[67,68] Maturo and colleagues[10] reported that children with VCD and GERD failed to improve on proton-pump inhibitor (PPI) therapy, but their VCD symptoms improved with speech therapy or psychiatric treatment. In their study of 62 subjects with VCD and GERD, Woolnough and colleagues[69] found that only 24.2% of adult patients reported improvement in VCD symptoms after 8-week treatment with PPI therapy twice daily. In a retrospective uncontrolled case series of 62 patients (aged 18–90 years) with confirmed VCD, low-dose amitriptyline at bedtime was beneficial in 90% of cases.[70]

As discussed previously, there seems to be an appreciable overlap between VCD and chronic refractory cough derived from laryngeal hypersensitivity studies. Gabapentin and speech therapy are recommended in the treatment of chronic unexplained cough.[71] One could review the findings from this sizable literature and potentially draw therapeutic conclusions relevant to VCD. However, clinicians should note that all studies were performed in adults only. The pediatric cough guidelines in children less than 14 years of age are dissimilar from the adult cough guidelines and do not address the concept of laryngeal hypersensitivity.[72]

FUTURE DIRECTIONS

Although significant progress has been achieved in our understanding of VCD, we are still in the early phases. The "hot" interconnectivity spot of upper and lower airways, brain activation centers, and gastrointestinal system resides in the larynx. The mechanisms underpinning the interplay between the structural elements, neurologic pathways, and inflammatory signals in the upper airway remain to be elucidated. Further phenotyping of patients and randomized clinical trials with quantifiable outcomes are necessary to advance the field of vocal cord dysfunction.

ACKNOWLEDGMENTS

Dr Petrov would like to extend his deep gratitude to Dr Rachel Schreiber for her meticulous editing of the article.

REFERENCES

1. Christopher KL, Wood RP 2nd, Eckert RC, et al. Vocal-cord dysfunction presenting as asthma. N Engl J Med 1983;308(26):1566–70.
2. Morris MJ, Christopher KL. Diagnostic criteria for the classification of vocal cord dysfunction. Chest 2010;138(5):1213–23.
3. Christensen PM, Heimdal JH, Christopher KL, et al. ERS/ELS/ACCP 2013 international consensus conference nomenclature on inducible laryngeal obstructions. Eur Respir Rev 2015;24(137):445–50.
4. Bardin PG, Low K, Ruane L, et al. Controversies and conundrums in vocal cord dysfunction. Lancet Respir Med 2017;5(7):546–8.
5. Bisdorff B, Kenn K, Nowak D, et al. Asthma and vocal cord dysfunction related symptoms in the general population—a pilot study. Ann Allergy Asthma Immunol 2014;113(5):576–7.
6. Morris MJ, Allan PF, Perkins PJ. Vocal cord dysfunction: etiologies and treatment. Clin Pulm Med 2006;13(2):73–86.
7. Brugman S. The many faces of vocal cord dysfunction: what 36 years of literature tell us. Am J Respir Crit Care Med 2003;167(7):A588.
8. Johansson H, Norlander K, Berglund L, et al. Prevalence of exercise-induced bronchoconstriction and exercise-induced laryngeal obstruction in a general adolescent population. Thorax 2015;70(1):57–63.
9. Christensen PM, Thomsen SF, Rasmussen N, et al. Exercise-induced laryngeal obstructions: prevalence and symptoms in the general public. Eur Arch Otorhinolaryngol 2011;268(9):1313.
10. Maturo S, Hill C, Bunting G, et al. Pediatric paradoxical vocal-fold motion: presentation and natural history. Pediatrics 2011;128:e1443–9.
11. Hseu A, Sandler M, Ericson D, et al. Paradoxical vocal fold motion in children presenting with exercise induced dyspnea. Int J Pediatr Otorhinolaryngol 2016;90: 165–9.
12. Traister RS, Fajt ML, Whitman-Purves E, et al. A retrospective analysis comparing subjects with isolated and coexistent vocal cord dysfunction and asthma. Allergy Asthma Proc 2013;34(4):349–55.
13. Fowler SJ, Thurston A, Chesworth B, et al. The VCDQ–a Questionnaire for symptom monitoring in vocal cord dysfunction. Clin Exp Allergy 2015;45(9):1406–11.
14. Dunglison RD. The practice of medicine. Philadelphia: Lea and Blanchard; 1842. p. 257–8.
15. Leo RJ, Konakanchi R. Psychogenic respiratory distress: a case of paradoxical vocal cord dysfunction and literature review. Prim Care Companion J Clin Psychiatry 1999;1(2):39.
16. Staudenmayer H, Christopher KL, Repsher L, et al. Mass psychogenic illness: psychological predisposition and iatrogenic pseudo-vocal cord dysfunction

and pseudo-reactive airways disease syndrome. J Med Toxicol 2011;7(2): 109–17.

17. Morris MJ, Oleszewski RT, Sterner JB, et al. Vocal cord dysfunction related to combat deployment. Mil Med 2013;178(11):1208–12.

18. Powell DM, Karanfilov BI, Beechler KB, et al. Paradoxical vocal cord dysfunction in juveniles. Arch Otolaryngol Head Neck Surg 2000;126(1):29–34.

19. Olin JT, Westhoff E. Exercise-induced laryngeal obstruction and performance psychology: using the mind as a diagnostic and therapeutic target. Immunol Allergy Clin N Am 2018;38:303–15.

20. Dietrich M, Andreatta RD, Jiang Y, et al. Preliminary findings on the relation between the personality trait of stress reaction and the central neural control of human vocalization. Int J Speech Lang Pathol 2012;14(4):377–89.

21. Kryshtopava M, Van Lierde K, Meerschman I, et al. Brain activity during phonation in women with muscle tension dysphonia: an fMRI study. J Voice 2017; 31(6):675–90.

22. Morrison M, Rammage L, Emami AJ. The irritable larynx syndrome. J Voice 1999; 13(3):447–55.

23. Vertigan AE, Bone SL, Gibson PG. Laryngeal sensory dysfunction in laryngeal hypersensitivity syndrome. Respirology 2013;18(6):948–56.

24. Ayres JG, Gabbott PL. Vocal cord dysfunction and laryngeal hyperresponsiveness: a function of altered autonomic balance? Thorax 2002;57(4):284–5.

25. Vertigan AE, Kapela SM, Kearney EK, et al. Laryngeal dysfunction in cough hypersensitivity syndrome: a cross-sectional observational study. J Allergy Clin Immunol Pract 2018;6(6):2087–95.

26. Gurevich-Uvena J, Parker JM, Fitzpatrick TM, et al. Medical comorbidities for paradoxical vocal fold motion (vocal cord dysfunction) in the military population. J Voice 2010;24(6):728–31.

27. Smith B, Milstein C, Rolfes B, et al. Paradoxical vocal fold motion (PVFM) in pediatric otolaryngology. Am J Otolaryngol 2017;38(2):230–2.

28. Peters EJ, Hatley TK, Crater SE, et al. Sinus computed tomography scan and markers of inflammation in vocal cord dysfunction and asthma. Ann Allergy Asthma Immunol 2003;90(3):316–22.

29. Forrest LA, Husein T, Husein O. Paradoxical vocal cord motion: classification and treatment. Laryngoscope 2012;122(4):844–53.

30. Patel DA, Blanco M, Vaezi MF. Laryngopharyngeal reflux and functional laryngeal disorder: perspective and common practice of the general gastroenterologist. Gastroenterol Hepatol 2018;14(9):512.

31. Marcinow AM, Thompson J, Forrest LA, et al. Irritant-induced paradoxical vocal fold motion disorder: diagnosis and management. Otolaryngol Head Neck Surg 2015;153(6):996–1000.

32. Anderson JA. Work-associated irritable larynx syndrome. Curr Opin Allergy Clin Immunol 2015;15(2):150–5.

33. Liyanagedara S, McLeod R, Elhassan HA. Exercise induced laryngeal obstruction: a review of diagnosis and management. Eur Arch Otorhinolaryngol 2017; 274(4):1781–9.

34. Røksund OD, Maat RC, Heimdal JH, et al. Exercise induced dyspnea in the young. Larynx as the bottleneck of the airways. Respir Med 2009;103(12): 1911–8.

35. Rundell KW, Spiering BA. Inspiratory stridor in elite athletes. Chest 2003;123(2): 468–74.

36. Maat RC, Hilland M, Røksund OD, et al. Exercise-induced laryngeal obstruction: natural history and effect of surgical treatment. Eur Arch Otorhinolaryngol 2011; 268(10):1485.

37. Perello MM, Gurevich J, Fitzpatrick T, et al. Clinical characteristics of vocal cord dysfunction in two military tertiary care facilities. Am J Respir Crit Care Med 2003; 167(suppl):A788.

38. Chiang T, Marcinow AM, deSilva BW, et al. Exercise-induced paradoxical vocal fold motion disorder: diagnosis and management. Laryngoscope 2013;123(3): 727–31.

39. Newman KB, Mason UG 3rd, Schmaling KB. Clinical features of vocal cord dysfunction. Am J Respir Crit Care Med 1995;152:1382–6.

40. Olin JT, Clary MS, Fan EM, et al. Continuous laryngoscopy quantitates laryngeal behaviour in exercise and recovery. Eur Respir J 2016;48(4):1192–200.

41. Olin JT, Clary MS, Connors D, et al. Glottic configuration in patients with exercise-induced stridor: a new paradigm. Laryngoscope 2014;124(11):2568–73.

42. Tervonen H, Niskanen MM, Sovijärvi AR, et al. Fiberoptic videolaryngoscopy during bicycle ergometry: A diagnostic tool for exercise-induced vocal cord dysfunction. Laryngoscope 2009;119(9):1776–80.

43. Hull JH, Walsted ES, Backer V, et al. High prevalence of laryngeal obstruction during exercise in severe asthma. Am J Respir Crit Care Med 2019;199(4): 538–42.

44. Low K, Lau KK, Holmes P, et al. Abnormal vocal cord function in difficult-to-treat asthma. Am J Respir Crit Care Med 2011;184(1):50–6.

45. Jain S, Bandi V, Zimmerman J, et al. Incidence of vocal cord dysfunction in patients presenting to emergency room with acute asthma exacerbation. Chest 1999;116(4):243S.

46. Traister RS, Fajt ML, Petrov AA. The morbidity and cost of vocal cord dysfunction misdiagnosed as asthma. Allergy Asthma Proc 2016;37(2):25–31.

47. Fajt ML, Traister RS, Petrov AA. Vocal cord dysfunction and asthma. Curr Treat Options Allergy 2017;4(3):329–41.

48. Nolan PK, Chrysler M, Phillips G, et al. Pulse oximetry coupled with spirometry in the emergency department helps differentiate an asthma exacerbation from possible vocal cord dysfunction. Pediatr Pulmonol 2007;42(7):605–9.

49. Watson MA, King CS, Holley AB, et al. Clinical and lung-function variables associated with vocal cord dysfunction. Respir Care 2009;54(4):467–73.

50. Nielsen EW, Hull JH, Backer V. High prevalence of exercise-induced laryngeal obstruction in athletes. Med Sci Sports Exerc 2013;45(11):2030–5.

51. Hull JH, Backer V, Gibson PG, et al. Laryngeal dysfunction: assessment and management for the clinician. Am J Respir Crit Care Med 2016;194(9):1062–72.

52. Traister RS, Fajt ML, Landsittel D, et al. A novel scoring system to distinguish vocal cord dysfunction from asthma. J Allergy Clin Immunol In Pract 2014; 2(1):65–9.

53. Barker N, Everard ML. Getting to grips with 'dysfunctional breathing'. Paediatr Respir Rev 2015;16(1):53–61.

54. Traister RS, Stoltz LP, Fajt ML, et al. Vocal cord dysfunction in patients with predominant upper airway symptoms. J Allergy Clin Immunol 2019;143(2):AB197.

55. Owens G, Petrov A. Successful desensitization of three patients with hypersensitivity reactions to omalizumab. Curr Drug Saf 2011;6(5):339–42.

56. Garcia-Neuer M, Lynch DM, Marquis K, et al. Drug-induced paradoxical vocal fold motion. J Allergy Clin Immunol In Pract 2018;6(1):90–4.

57. Fajt ML, Rosenberg SL, Yecies E, et al. A 10-year experience of a novel and safe modified environmental rush immunotherapy protocol. Allergy Asthma Proc 2017; 38:4.
58. Fajt ML, Birnie KM, Bittar HE, et al. Co-existence of vocal cord dysfunction with pulmonary conditions other than asthma: a case series. Respir Med case Rep 2018;25:104–8.
59. Denipah N, Dominguez CM, Kraai EP, et al. Acute management of paradoxical vocal fold motion (vocal cord dysfunction). Ann Emerg Med 2017;69(1):18–23.
60. Shaffer M, Litts JK, Nauman E, et al. Speech-language pathology as a primary treatment for exercise-induced laryngeal obstruction. Immunol Allergy Clin North Am 2018;38(2):293–302.
61. Patel RR, Venediktov R, Schooling T, et al. Evidence-based systematic review: effects of speech-language pathology treatment for individuals with paradoxical vocal fold motion. Am J Speech Lang Pathol 2015;24(3):566–84.
62. Drake K, Palmer AD, Schindler JS, et al. Functional outcomes after behavioral treatment of paradoxical vocal fold motion in adults. Folia Phoniatr Logop 2017; 69(4):154–68.
63. Doshi DR, Weinberger MM. Long-term outcome of vocal cord dysfunction. Ann Allergy Asthma Immunol 2006;96(6):794–9.
64. Hynes G, Bakere H, McAleer C, et al. The benefits of an integrated vocal cord dysfunction service in treating a subgroup of patients with difficult to control asthma. Am J Respir Crit Care Med 2015;191:A3813.
65. Kramer S, deSilva B, Forrest LA, et al. Does treatment of paradoxical vocal fold movement disorder decrease asthma medication use? Laryngoscope 2017; 127(7):1531–7.
66. Guglani L, Atkinson S, Hosanagar A, et al. A systematic review of psychological interventions for adult and pediatric patients with vocal cord dysfunction. Front Pediatr 2014;2:82.
67. Denoyelle F, Garabedian EN, Roger G, et al. Laryngeal dyskinesia as a cause of stridor in infants. Arch Otolaryngol Head Neck Surg 1996;122(6):612–6.
68. Ferster AP, Shokri T, Carr M. Diagnosis and treatment of paradoxical vocal fold motion in infants. Int J Pediatr Otorhinolaryngol 2018;107:6–9.
69. Woolnough K, Blakey J, Pargeter N, et al. Acid suppression does not reduce symptoms from vocal cord dysfunction, where gastro-laryngeal reflux is a known trigger. Respirology 2013;18(3):553–4.
70. Varney VA, Parnell H, Evans J, et al. The successful treatment of vocal cord dysfunction with low-dose amitriptyline–including literature review. Journal of asthma and allergy 2009;2:105.
71. Gibson P, Wang G, McGarvey L, et al. Treatment of unexplained chronic cough: CHEST guideline and expert panel report. Chest 2016;149(1):27–44.
72. Chang AB, Oppenheimer JJ, Weinberger M, et al. Etiologies of chronic cough in pediatric cohorts: CHEST guideline and expert panel report. Chest 2017;152(3): 607–17.

It's Time to Start Phenotyping Our Patients with Asthma

Hannah Duffey, MD, William C. Anderson III, MD*

KEYWORDS

- Asthma • Biologic • Biomarker • Controller • Endotype • Management • Pediatric
- Phenotype

KEY POINTS

- Phenotyping pediatric patients with asthma could aid medical providers in assessing response to treatment and difficulty in gaining asthma control, predicting asthma development, and initiating or stepping-up controller therapy.
- Phenotyping can be done in the clinic using demographics and readily attainable biomarkers including IgE, skin prick testing, ImmunoCAP testing, fractional exhaled nitric oxide, and spirometry.
- The development of biologic therapies for asthma emphasize the importance of phenotyping, especially when deciding which biologic to select and predicting response to therapy.

INTRODUCTION

The advent of new therapies, ranging from inhaled corticosteroids (ICS) to biologics, has led to advances in the management of pediatric patients with asthma. These therapies offer practitioners the ability to provide tailored, precision treatments to individual patients, thereby targeting therapies based on likelihood of response, reducing unnecessary or potentially harmful interventions, and minimizing side effects. Despite these advances, asthma treatment guidelines are lagging behind these advancements, leaving providers with limited guidance of which new therapeutic is best for their patients, especially for pediatric patients.

Precision medicine has been defined as targeted therapies based on genetic, biomarker, phenotypic, or psychosocial features differentiating an individual patient from another.[1] Precision medicine distinguishes a specific patient from others with

Disclosure Statement: Dr H. Duffey has nothing to disclose. Dr W.C. Anderson served on an advisory board for AstraZeneca.
Department of Pediatrics, Division of Allergy and Immunology, Children's Hospital Colorado, University of Colorado School of Medicine, 13123 East 16th Avenue, Box 518, Aurora, CO 80045, USA
* Corresponding author.
E-mail address: william.anderson@childrenscolorado.org

a similar or even the same presentation. Although arguably precision medicine has existed for a long time, the rapid rate of diagnostic and therapeutic advances is allowing caregivers to provide even more individualized therapy plans than were previously available. Precision medicine is being used routinely in many fields of medicine. The discovery of estrogen receptor expression in certain forms of breast cancer led to the development of selective estrogen receptor modulators for those with estrogen receptor–positive breast cancer.[2] The understanding of genetic abnormalities leading to different defects in the protein structure of cystic fibrosis transmembrane conductance regulator led to the advent of ivacaftor and lumacaftor to treat patients with cystic fibrosis who have specific genetic mutations.[3]

Current asthma management is based on avoidance of known triggers and the use of a variety of controller medications including ICS, long-acting beta agonists (LABAs), leukotriene receptor antagonists (LTRAs), and now most recently multiple biologics, targeting the mechanisms of T_H2 inflammation. Using precision medicine to select the correct therapy for individual patients could both improve day-to-day asthma control and reduce exacerbations while decreasing health care costs and decreasing the side effects from unnecessary medications. Attempting to identify biomarkers to better understand a patient's underlying disease process is critical to selecting new treatments. Only recently, the Global Initiative for Asthma has embarked on this endeavor of precision medicine by providing guidance on biologic choice for severe asthma based on specific biomarkers identified from clinical trials.[4] This review is intended to highlight the importance of phenotyping pediatric patients with asthma to provide an individualized approach to care.

BIOMARKERS, PHENOTYPES, AND ENDOTYPES

Asthma is a heterogenous condition involving an array of underlying mechanisms that ultimately result in inflammation of the airways and present as reversible airway obstruction. Phenotypes and endotypes have been used to try to better categorize patients and understand their underlying mechanisms for disease. Phenotypes are observable characteristics or outward manifestations of underlying genetics and pathophysiology.[5] Endotypes further subtype phenotypes based on pathophysiologic mechanisms underlying the disease process.[5] A phenotype–endotype association in asthma is exemplified in aspirin-exacerbated respiratory disease. Aspirin-exacerbated respiratory disease has an underlying pathophysiologic mechanism involving an upregulation in leukotriene production, leading to a clinical presentation including asthma, sinusitis with nasal polyposis, and sensitivity to nonsteroidal anti-inflammatory drugs.

The distinctions of phenotypes have frequently been made through the use of biomarkers. The ideal biomarker is readily available, easily interpretable, minimally invasive, and reproducible over time.[6] Various phenotypic markers used in classifying patients with asthma have included demographics such as race, blood eosinophil levels, periostin, fractional exhaled nitric oxide (F_ENO), aeroallergen skin prick testing or ImmunoCAP, and serum IgE (**Box 1**). In the pediatric asthma population, most biomarkers to date have been associated with T_H2 inflammation, in particular F_ENO, sensitization to aeroallergens by skin prick testing, IgE levels, and serum eosinophils. Biomarkers have been examined in the context of predicting development of asthma in children,[7] exacerbation rates,[8] difficulty in gaining control,[9] and response to therapy.[10–12]

The following sections highlight examples of how the practicing clinician can use asthma phenotypes and biomarkers to provide tailored therapy for their patients.

Box 1
Clinical variables and biomarkers used to phenotype pediatric asthma

- Aeroallergen skin prick testing/ImmunoCAP
- Total IgE
- Blood eosinophil count
- $F_E NO$
- Spirometry with bronchodilator response
- Rhinitis symptoms
- Demographic features including race and body mass index

PHENOTYPING PATIENTS TO DETERMINE ASTHMA SEVERITY

Multiple studies have sought to better define asthmatic phenotypes with the goal of identifying patient characteristics that may predict response to various therapies. An initial cluster analysis in adults with obstructive airway diseases identified specific phenotypes suggesting an alternate management strategy based on patient characteristics, which deviated from current guidelines.[13,14] This finding led to several studies that examined children with asthma and attempted to better define underlying phenotypes (**Table 1**). Similar to the adult studies, children were grouped into clusters with phenotypic characteristics focused primarily on atopy, airway physiology, symptom onset, and asthma symptom days and exacerbations.[15–18]

In a study by Fitzpatrick and colleagues,[15] cluster analysis similar to that used in the adult Severe Asthma Research Program identified four clusters of patients. Cluster 1 children had relatively normal lung function and less atopy.[15] Cluster 2 children had slightly lower lung function and increased atopy, symptoms, and medication use.[15] Cluster 3 children had more comorbidities such as gastroesophageal reflux disease and chronic sinusitis, lower lung function, and increased bronchial hyperresponsiveness.[15] Cluster 4 consisted of children with the lowest lung function and greatest symptoms and medication use.[15] Chang and colleagues[18] performed a cluster analysis in the population of children who participated in the Childhood Asthma Research and Education network clinical trials. Four clusters of pediatric patients were identified that were similar to the Severe Asthma Research Program children. Howrylak and colleagues[16] used patients from the Childhood Asthma Management Program, which represented patients with more mild to moderate asthma, and defined 5 different clusters of patients based on atopy, airway physiology, and exacerbations, with differences in the more severe clusters based on their responses to ICS and nedocromil.

Most recently, Zoratti and colleagues[17] examined a population participating in the Inner City Asthma Consortium to define 5 different clusters (clusters A–E) of children based on blood eosinophilia, total IgE, allergic sensitization, $F_E NO$, pulmonary physiology, and degree of asthma and rhinitis symptoms. The majority of the most symptomatic patients had the most allergic phenotype; however, a smaller subset of children with relatively little allergic inflammation also were identified who were symptomatic.[17] Cluster E was identified as the most symptomatic, unresponsive to therapy, and also had the highest levels of markers of $T_H 2$ inflammation, suggesting that this group may be the subset who would benefit most from newer biologic medications.[17] Similarly, Pongracic and colleagues[9] used the Inner City Asthma Consortium population to identify those patients who would have difficult-to-control asthma, as defined by higher doses of ICS with or without LABA. The baseline forced expiratory volume in

Table 1
Summary of pediatric asthma phenotype cluster analyses

Reference	Population	Age (y)	Number of Patients	Phenotypic Variables	Description of Clusters
Fitzpatrick et al,[15] 2011	Persistent asthma recruited from 4 academic centers in the United States	6–17	161	Pulmonary physiology Markers of allergic sensitization and inflammation (F_ENO, SPT, total serum IgE, and serum eosinophils Asthma history and control	Cluster 1: Late-onset ($\sim$2–10 y old) symptomatic asthma with normal lung function Cluster 2: Early-onset (1 mo–5 y old) atopic asthma with normal lung function Cluster 3: Early-onset (2 mo–2.5 y old) atopic asthma with mild airflow limitation Cluster 4: Early-onset (2 mo–3 y old) atopic asthma with advanced airflow limitation
Zoratti et al,[17] 2016	Persistent asthma recruited from low-income areas in 9 US cities	6–17	717	Pulmonary physiology Markers of allergic sensitization and inflammation (F_ENO, SPT, total serum IgE and eosinophils) Asthma history and control Rhinitis severity	Cluster A: minimally symptomatic asthma and rhinitis, lower allergy and inflammation, and normal pulmonary physiology Cluster B: highly symptomatic asthma despite high step-level treatment, intermediate rhinitis, lower allergy and inflammation, and mildly altered pulmonary physiology Cluster C: minimally symptomatic asthma and rhinitis, intermediate allergy and inflammation, and mildly impaired pulmonary physiology Clusters D: minimally symptomatic asthma, intermediate rhinitis, higher levels of allergy and allergic inflammation, and an intermediate degree of pulmonary physiology Cluster E: most symptomatic asthma and rhinitis while receiving high step-level treatment and had the highest total serum IgE level, blood eosinophil count, and allergen sensitizations

Source	Age	N	Parameters	Clusters
Howrylak et al,[16] 2014	5–12	1041	Pulmonary physiology Atopic history Markers of allergic sensitization and inflammation (SPT, total serum IgE and eosinophils) Asthma history (specifically exacerbation risk)	Cluster 1: Mild asthma with low atopy, obstruction and exacerbation rate Cluster 2: Atopic asthma with low levels of obstruction and medium rates of exacerbation Cluster 3: Atopic asthma with high levels of obstruction and medium rates of exacerbation Cluster 4: Moderately atopic asthma with high levels of obstruction and high exacerbation rates Cluster 5: Highly atopic asthma with high levels of obstruction and high exacerbation rates
			Mild to moderate persistent asthma recruited from the Childhood Asthma Management Program	
Chang et al,[18] 2014	6–18	611	Pulmonary physiology Markers of allergic sensitization and inflammation (F_ENO, SPT, total serum IgE and eosinophils) Asthma history and control Comorbidities	Cluster 1: Late onset (~3–8 y old), normal lung function, lowest F_ENO and IgE Cluster 2: Early onset (~2 mo–2 y old), normal lung function Cluster 3: Early onset (~4 mo–2 y old), higher comorbid conditions Cluster 4: Early onset (~2 mo–3 y old), impaired lung function
			Mild to moderate persistent asthma recruited from Childhood Asthma Research and Education network clinical trials	

Abbreviation: SPT, skin prick testing.

1 second (FEV$_1$) bronchodilator responsiveness was the most important distinguishing characteristic, followed by markers of rhinitis severity and atopy.[9]

These studies illustrate that, by obtaining baseline biomarkers in patients with persistent asthma, clinicians may more readily identify those patients who are at increased risk for difficult-to-control and severe asthma, despite good adherence to standard guideline therapy. These patients may benefit from more frequent symptom monitoring, increased identification of triggers, patient education, and potentially targeted use of biologic therapies.

PREDICTING ASTHMA DEVELOPMENT IN YOUNG CHILDREN

The diagnosis of asthma in young children and the differentiation of which children may go on to develop asthma is an important question for both parents and clinicians. Typical testing such as spirometry could be attempted if you have a cooperative child nearing school age, but this modality does not help in a younger population. Anderson and colleagues[7] demonstrated that biomarkers can aid physicians in determining which children will go on to develop asthma. They followed 244 children from birth and collected blood samples at 2, 4, 6, and 11 years of age to assess the relationships among aeroallergen sensitization, blood eosinophils, and periostin levels with the development of asthma.[7] Aeroallergen sensitization, and eosinophilia were found to be predictors of asthma development in young children.[7] Periostin was not found to be helpful given bone turnover in children, which can result in elevated periostin.[7] Aeroallergen sensitization and eosinophil levels meet the aforementioned qualities of a good biomarker and importantly are easily obtainable in young children. Such testing would be beneficial to obtain in toddlers and preschool-aged children with recurrent wheezing to help guide future management and help families to anticipate their children's future care.

SELECTING CONTROLLER AND STEP-UP THERAPIES

The management of asthma for the past decade has been guided by the National, Heart, Lung and Blood Institute (NHLBI) Expert Panel 3 from 2007.[19] In this report, biomarkers were discussed with respect to management; however, patient phenotypes were not taken into account in the creation of the stepwise approach to management. The traditional stepwise approach for asthma management is helpful, but with the advances in available therapies, we need an updated approach, incorporating patient phenotypes and endotypes into diagnostic and management decisions.

The initiation of asthma therapy in the very young population can be challenging for providers and parents, particularly given concerns for medication side effects in these patients, including a decrease in linear growth associated with ICSs.[20] The Individualized Therapy for Asthma in Toddlers study examined response to daily ICS, as needed ICS, and LTRA based on phenotyping in children 12 to 59 month old.[21] Children with peripheral blood eosinophil counts of 300 cells/μL or greater and aeroallergen sensitization had better responses to daily ICS therapy with fewer exacerbations and more asthma control days than other therapies.[21] Overall, children requiring the initiation of asthma therapy responded the best to daily ICS therapy, but the subset with the presence of these biomarkers derived the greatest benefit.[21] In the patient group that had no aeroallergen sensitization and with peripheral blood eosinophil counts of less than 300 cells/μL, there was no difference in their response to daily ICS, as-needed ICS, or LTRA.[21]

In a study by Szefler and colleagues,[10] the responses to ICS and LTRA in 6- to 17-year-old patients with mild to moderate persistent asthma were compared. ICS were superior to LTRA in patients with evidence of allergic inflammation, including elevated $F_E NO$, eosinophilia, and elevated IgE levels.[10] Those with lower lung function and a lower methacholine PC_{20} also responded better to ICS.[10] Meanwhile, the authors suggested that patients with normal lung function and no evidence of allergic inflammation could be trialed on either ICS or LTRA.[10] The use of $F_E NO$ as a biomarker for medication selection has been validated in additional pediatric studies. Pediatric patients with asthma and elevated $F_E NO$ have been shown to have more asthma control days when treated with ICS.[22] $F_E NO$ can be used by practitioners to determine the likelihood of response to ICS and for the monitoring of compliance with ICS therapy.[11]

Biomarkers can be useful in guiding the appropriate step-up treatment for pediatric patients with uncontrolled asthma. The Best Add-on Therapy Giving Effective Response (BADGER) study found overall that LABAs were the most effective step up therapy compared with increased ICS dosing or addition of LTRA for 6- to 17-year-old children with uncontrolled asthma on low-dose ICSs.[23] A post hoc analysis of the BADGER study demonstrated differences in response to add-on therapy based on a history of eczema and patient race.[24] In patients without eczema regardless of ethnicity, the addition of LABA was superior to the other therapies.[24] In those with eczema, the best response to step-up therapy was dependent on ethnicity, with black children responding best to increased ICS, white Hispanic children responding best to LTRA addition, and white non-Hispanic children responding best to either LABA or LTRA addition.[24]

SELECTING A BIOLOGIC

The advent of multiple biologics for the management of severe asthma in pediatric and adolescent patients highlight the imperative to phenotype our patients to provide targeted care. These therapies are ideal in the field of precision medicine given their degree of specificity to target a specific cytokine, antibody, or receptor. Given the financial and time costs to patients for these biologics, as well as their relatively more invasive administration compared with other controller therapies, identifying which patients are best suited for each therapy before initiation would be ideal. Biologic medications currently possessing an approval from the US Food and Drug Administration for pediatric and adolescent patients include omalizumab, mepolizumab, benralizumab, and dupilumab, all of which focus on T_H2-mediated inflammation (**Table 2**). At the time of publication, resilizumab was only approved for adults. With the exception of omalizumab, most studies to date have only included patients as young as 12 years old, and even then that adolescent population was not robustly represented in the trials, emphasizing the need for pediatric specific trials.

Omalizumab

The benefits of omalizumab in asthma have been well-established, including reduced exacerbations, symptoms, health care use, missed school days, and oral corticosteroid use.[25] In inner-city patients with asthma aged 6 to 20 years with persistent or uncontrolled asthma, the addition of omalizumab to NHLBI guideline-based therapy reduced symptom days, exacerbations, and ICS dose.[26] Notably, the additional of omalizumab reduced seasonal exacerbations in this treatment group compared with placebo.[26] A post hoc analysis examining the efficacy of omalizumab found participants with $F_E NO$ of 20 ppb or greater, blood eosinophils of 2% or greater, and a body mass index of 25 or greater were more likely to benefit with respect to reduced exacerbations.[27] Beyond these biomarkers, prior exacerbations and NHLBI controller step therapy has been identified as phenotypic predictors of omalizumab response in

Table 2
Summary of biologics approved for pediatric asthma

Biologic	Mechanism of Action	FDA Approval Age for Asthma	Indications	Dose, Route and Dosing Interval	Predictors of Response
Omalizumab	Humanized, monoclonal anti-IgE binding free IgE	≥6 y old	Moderate-to-severe persistent asthma, symptoms inadequately controlled with ICS, perennial aeroallergen sensitization	Based on age, weight, and IgE levels; SQ	Elevated F$_E$NO Elevated serum eosinophils Body mass index of ≥25 Exacerbations on NHLBI Step 5 therapy
Mepolizumab	Humanized, monoclonal antibody binding to IL-5	≥12 y old	Severe persistent asthma, eosinophilic phenotype	100 mg SQ every 4 wk	Elevated serum eosinophils Frequent exacerbations
Benralizumab	Humanized, monoclonal antibody against the IL-5α receptor leading to antibody-dependent cell-mediated cytotoxicity	≥12 y old	Severe persistent asthma, eosinophilic phenotype	30 mg SQ every 4 wk for the first 3 doses then spaced to every 8 wk thereafter	Elevated serum eosinophils Frequent exacerbations
Dupilumab	Fully humanized, monoclonal antibody against the IL-4 α receptor blocking both the IL-4 and IL-13 pathways	≥12 y old	Moderate-to-severe persistent asthma, eosinophilic phenotype, or with oral corticosteroid dependent asthma	Initial dose: 400 mg or 600 mg SQ Maintenance dose: 200 mg or 300 mg SQ every 2 wk	Elevated serum eosinophils Frequent exacerbations Elevated F$_E$NO

Abbreviation: SQ, subcutaneous.

pediatric patients. In the Preventative Omalizumab or Step-Up Therapy for Fall Exacerbations, Teach and colleagues[28] found those pediatric patients on NHLBI treatment step 5 and who had an exacerbation in the run-in period had the greatest reduction in fall exacerbations with the addition of omalizumab.

Mepolizumab

Mepolizumab has been found to reduce exacerbations, hospitalizations, and emergency room visits, while increasing the time to first exacerbations and improving pre-bronchodilator and post-bronchodilator FEV_1.[29,30] Of note, these findings were only found when the patient population was selected for signs of eosinophilic inflammation including peripheral blood eosinophilia, sputum eosinophilia, and elevated F_ENO.[29,30] Adolescents 12 years and older were included in both of these studies, but their numbers were relatively small compared with adult patients and no specific studies looking at a pediatric population have been published at this time. Pediatric specific studies must be performed as currently we can only extrapolate data from these adolescent and adult studies. Among adult patients, an elevated blood eosinophil count and increased exacerbation in the prior year were the greatest predictors for a decrease in exacerbations with mepolizumab.[29]

Benralizumab

Benralizumab has been demonstrated to reduce exacerbations, improve symptoms, and increase pre-bronchodilator FEV_1 in adolescent and adult patients who were not well-controlled despite medium- to high-dose ICS/LABA therapy compared with placebo.[31,32] Of note in both of these studies the adolescent population accounted for only a small proportion of the total study population in the final analysis at approximately 5.2% and 2.4%.[31,32] In a study combining 2 phase III trials, the researchers concluded that the extent to which exacerbation rates were decreased with benralizumab increased with increasing blood eosinophil counts and in patients with higher rates of exacerbation.[33] The studies examined patients with peripheral blood eosinophils 300 cells/μL or greater and those with less than 300 cells/μL.[33]

Dupilumab

In a study assessing efficacy and safety, dupilumab decreased exacerbation rates in patients 12 years of age or older with uncontrolled asthma and improved FEV_1 by 0.32 L compared with 0.14 L with placebo.[34] The annual rate of exacerbation was decreased even further in patients with an absolute eosinophil counts 300 cells/mm^3 or greater, whereas those with an eosinophil count of less than 150/mm^3 had no significant difference in exacerbation rates between the dupilumab and placebo groups.[34] Additionally, patients with elevated F_ENO showed greater benefit with respect to reduction in exacerbations.[34] In this study again only approximately 5.6% of participants were adolescents.[34] In another study examining the impact of dupilumab in reducing oral glucocorticoid doses in patients with glucocorticoid-dependent asthma, the researchers found a reduction in glucocorticoid dose regardless of eosinophil count, but found a greater impact on those with peripheral blood eosinophil counts of 300/mm^3 or greater.[35]

SUMMARY

The evidence for asthma management has advanced such that the use of basic screening biomarkers, including IgE, eosinophil counts, and aeroallergen sensitization, for pediatric patients with asthma can provide tailored, personalized management. By phenotyping pediatric patients with asthma, health care providers can recognize which may be more difficult to treat, which may be more symptomatic or prone to exacerbations, and which may benefit from one controller therapy over another. As approval for biologics continue to move to younger populations, researchers should explore key phenotypic features that would identify which patients would best respond to one biologic over another. Future asthma management guidelines should incorporate this evidence to provide direction on which biologic or controller therapy should be chosen. Phenotyping pediatric patients with asthma will allow providers to elevate existing treatment strategies to provide precision care for their patients and hopefully improve outcomes.

REFERENCES

1. Jameson JL, Longo DL. Precision medicine — personalized, problematic, and promising. N Engl J Med 2015;372:2229–34.
2. Deluche E, Onesti CE, Andre F. Precision medicine for metastatic breast cancer. American Society for Clinical Oncology Educational Book; 2015. p. e2–7.
3. Rehman A. Lumacaftor–Ivacaftor in patients with cystic fibrosis homozygous for Phe508del CFTR. N Engl J Med 2015;373:1783–4.
4. Global Initiative for Asthma. Difficult-to-treat and severe asthma in adolescents and adult patients. A GINA pocket guide for health professionals. 2018. Available at: https://ginasthma.org/severeasthma2018/. Accessed February 16, 2019.
5. Skloot SG. Asthma phenotypes and endotypes: a personalized approach to treatment. Curr Opin Pulm Med 2016;22:3–9.
6. Anderson WC 3rd, Szefler SJ. Controlling the risk domain in pediatric asthma through personalized care. Semin Respir Crit Care Med 2018;39:36–44.
7. Anderson HM, Lemanske RF, Arron JR, et al. Relationships among aeroallergen sensitization, peripheral blood eosinophils, and periostin in pediatric asthma development. J Allergy Clin Immunol 2017;139:790–6.
8. Petsky HL, Kew KM, Chang AB. Exhaled nitric oxide levels to guide treatment for children with asthma. Cochrane Database Syst Rev 2016;(11):CD011439.
9. Pongracic JA, Krouse RZ, Babineau DC, et al. Distinguishing characteristics of difficult-to-control asthma in inner-city children and adolescents. J Allergy Clin Immunol 2016;138:1030–41.
10. Szefler SJ, Phillips BR, Martinez FD, et al. Characterization of within-subject responses to fluticasone and montelukast in childhood asthma. J Allergy Clin Immunol 2005;115:233–42.
11. Dweik RA, Boggs PB, Erzurum SC, et al. An official ATS clinical practice guideline: interpretation of exhaled nitric oxide levels (FENO) for clinical applications. Am J Respir Crit Care Med 2011;184:602.
12. Cowan DC, Taylor DR, Peterson LE, et al. Biomarker-based asthma phenotypes of corticosteroid response. J Allergy Clin Immunol 2015;135:877–83.e1.
13. Weatherall M, Travers J, Shirtcliffe PM, et al. Distinct clinical phenotypes of airways disease defined by cluster analysis. Eur Respir J 2009;34:812.
14. Moore WC, Meyers DA, Wenzel SE, et al. Identification of asthma phenotypes using cluster analysis in the Severe Asthma Research Program. Am J Respir Crit Care Med 2010;181:315.
15. Fitzpatrick AM, Teague WG, Meyers DA, et al. Heterogeneity of severe asthma in childhood: confirmation by cluster analysis of children in the National Institutes of

Health/National Heart, Lung, and Blood Institute Severe Asthma Research Program. J Allergy Clin Immunol 2011;127:382–9.e13.

16. Howrylak JA, Fuhlbrigge AL, Strunk RC, et al. Classification of childhood asthma phenotypes and long-term clinical responses to inhaled anti-inflammatory medications. J Allergy Clin Immunol 2014;133:1289–300.

17. Zoratti EM, Krouse RZ, Babineau DC, et al. Asthma phenotypes in inner-city children. J Allergy Clin Immunol 2016;138:1016–29.

18. Chang TS, Lemanske RF, Mauger DT, et al. Childhood asthma clusters and response to therapy in clinical trials. J Allergy Clin Immunol 2014;133:363–9.e3.

19. National Asthma Education and Prevention Program. Expert Panel Report 3 (EPR-3): guidelines for the Diagnosis and Management of Asthma-Summary Report 2007. J Allergy Clin Immunol 2007;120:S94–138.

20. Kelly HW, Sternberg AL, Lescher R, et al. Effect of inhaled glucocorticoids in childhood on adult height. N Engl J Med 2012;367:904–12.

21. Fitzpatrick AM, Jackson DJ, Mauger DT, et al. Individualized therapy for persistent asthma in young children. J Allergy Clin Immunol 2016;138:1608–18.e12.

22. Knuffman JE, Sorkness CA, Lemanske RF, et al. Phenotypic predictors of long-term response to inhaled corticosteroid and leukotriene modifier therapies in pediatric asthma. J Allergy Clin Immunol 2009;123:411–6.

23. Lemanske RF, Mauger DT, Sorkness CA, et al. Step-up therapy for children with uncontrolled asthma receiving inhaled corticosteroids. N Engl J Med 2010;362:975–85.

24. Malka J, Mauger DT, Covar R, et al. Eczema and race as combined determinants for differential response to step-up asthma therapy. J Allergy Clin Immunol 2014;134:483–5.

25. Humbert M, Busse WW, Hanania NA, et al. Omalizumab in asthma: an updated on recent developments. J Allergy Clin Immunol Pract 2014;2:525–36.

26. Busse WW, Morgan WJ, Gergen PJ, et al. Randomized trial of omalizumab (Anti-IgE) for asthma in inner-city children. N Engl J Med 2011;364:1005–15.

27. Sorkness CA, Wildfire JJ, Calatroni A, et al. Reassessment of omalizumab-dosing strategies and pharmacodynamics in inner-city children and adolescents. J Allergy Clin Immunol Pract 2013;1:163.

28. Teach SJ, Gill MA, Togias A, et al. Preseasonal treatment with either omalizumab or an inhaled corticosteroid boost to prevent fall asthma exacerbations. J Allergy Clin Immunol 2015;136:1476–85.

29. Pavord ID, Korn S, Howarth P, et al. Mepolizumab for severe eosinophilic asthma (DREAM): a multicentre, double-blind, placebo-controlled trial. Lancet 2012;380:651–9.

30. Ortega HG, Liu MC, Pavord ID, et al. Mepolizumab treatment in patients with severe eosinophilic asthma. N Engl J Med 2014;371:1198–207.

31. Bleecker ER, Fitzgerald JM, Chanez P, et al. Efficacy and safety of benralizumab for patients with severe asthma uncontrolled with high-dosage inhaled corticosteroids and long-acting β2-agonists (SIROCCO): a randomised, multicentre, placebo-controlled phase 3 trial. Lancet 2016;388:2115–27.

32. FitzGerald JM, Bleecker ER, Nair P, et al. Benralizumab, an anti-interleukin-5 receptor α monoclonal antibody, as add-on treatment for patients with severe, uncontrolled, eosinophilic asthma (CALIMA): a randomised, double-blind, placebo-controlled phase 3 trial. Lancet 2016;388:2128–41.

33. Fitzgerald JM, Bleecker ER, Menzies-Gow A, et al. Predictors of enhanced response with benralizumab for patients with severe asthma: pooled analysis of the SIROCCO and CALIMA studies. Lancet Respir Med 2018;6:51–64.
34. Castro M, Corren J, Pavord ID, et al. Dupilumab efficacy and safety in moderate-to-severe uncontrolled asthma. N Engl J Med 2018;378:2486–96.
35. Rabe KF, Nair P, Brusselle G, et al. Efficacy and safety of dupilumab in glucocorticoid-dependent severe asthma. N Engl J Med 2018;378:2475–85.

Asthma Self-management
It's Not One Size Fits All

Lisa Ulrich, MD*, Sabrina Palacios, MD

KEYWORDS

- Asthma • Asthma exacerbation • Asthma self-management
- Asthma home management

KEY POINTS

- Asthma exacerbations are a significant cause of health care use.
- Home self-management of asthma exacerbations is possible and there are many treatment options available.
- An asthma home self-management therapy plan should be personalized for each patient.
- Continued research into best practices for home asthma management is needed.

INTRODUCTION

Asthma is one of the most common chronic health conditions, with an estimated 339 million people affected worldwide according to the Global Asthma Network.[1] In 2016 in the United States, 8.3% of both children and adults were affected. Asthma was in the top 20 leading primary diagnoses for emergency department visits with a total of 1.7 million visits reported in 2015.[2]

Asthma accounted for 3518 deaths in 2016 in the United States alone.[3] According to the Centers for Disease Control and Prevention (CDC), 46.9% of people with asthma have reported 1 or more asthma exacerbations in the last year.[3] Definitions for asthma exacerbations can vary but typically are characterized by an increase in asthma symptoms, increase in use of reliever medications, or a decrease in measured expiratory airflow.[4–6] Exacerbations can result in acute care visits but some can be successfully managed at home. Self-management interventions have been associated with decreased health care use and improved quality-of-life outcomes.[7] A written asthma action plan is essential for asthma self-management in exacerbations.[5,7] This article focuses on multiple medication options available for self-management of asthma exacerbations in the home setting (**Fig. 1**).

Disclosure: The authors have no financial disclosures.
Department of Pediatrics, Division of Pulmonary Medicine, Nationwide Children's Hospital, The Ohio State University College of Medicine, 700 Childrens Drive, Columbus, OH 43205, USA
* Corresponding author.
E-mail address: LISA.ULRICH@NATIONWIDECHILDRENS.ORG

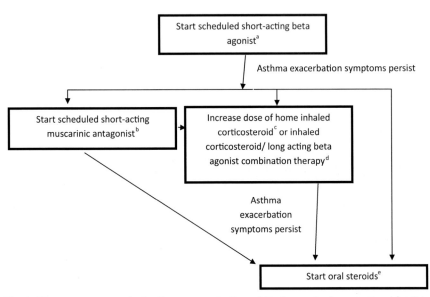

Fig. 1. Home management of asthma exacerbations. [a] Dosing varies by age. Consider 2 to 8 puffs with metered dose inhaler (MDI) with spacer or nebulizer treatment every 3 to 4 hours. [b] Dosing varies with age. Consider 2 puffs with MDI with spacer or nebulizer treatment every 6 hours. [c] Increase daily dose by 2 to 4 times. [d] Maximum dose suggested of 72 μg of formoterol in a day. [e] Dosing varies by age. In adults consider 1 mg/kg/d with maximum of 50 to 60 mg/d for 5 to 7 days. In children consider 1 to 2 mg/kg/d with maximum dosage of 40 to 60 mg/d for 3 to 5 days. There is no defined role for azithromycin, long-acting muscarinic antagonist, or leukotrienes in acute asthma exacerbations.

NONPHARMACOLOGIC INTERVENTIONS

Common sense and current Expert Panel Report 3 (EPR-3) guidelines suggest that removal of allergens and irritants should help in preventing asthma exacerbations.[4] This advice includes controlling common indoor allergens such as dust mites and indoor animal dander exposure, mold removal, and decreasing secondhand smoke exposure. Suggestions for allergen control include air purification, carpet removal, vacuuming using a high-efficiency particulate air–filtered machine, and use of dust mite repellant mattress covers or even acaricides to kill dust mites. In addition, removal of stuffed animals and house pets from the bedroom may help prevent allergen-related exacerbations.[4] However, a recent review of these interventions showed that although quality of life improved with a single intervention, it did not alter asthma-related health care use or lung function testing.[8] It is yet to be studied whether specific intervention combinations have more of an effect than others. Aside from the aforementioned exposures, β-blocker therapy and nonsteroidal antiinflammatory drug (NSAID) use should also be assessed to evaluate for nontraditional triggers and drug-drug interactions.[4]

It is well known that secondhand smoke exposure can lead to asthma exacerbations in both children and adults.[9] There are strong recommendations to avoid secondhand smoke exposure in the home and in the car, and to avoid personal use of cigarettes.[4] Not much is known about long-term exposure to electronic nicotine delivery systems (vaping). Early research suggests this environmental irritant may also be a trigger to asthma exacerbations and should be avoided, similar to conventional cigarette smoke.[10]

CLASSIC PHARMACOLOGIC INTERVENTIONS FOR ASTHMA EXACERBATION
Short-Acting Beta Agonist

Short-acting beta agonists (SABAs) (albuterol, salbutamol, and levalbuterol) work by binding to the beta-2 adrenergic receptors on small airway smooth muscle, leading to muscle relaxation and bronchodilation. Guidelines recommend early initiation of this therapy in asthma exacerbations.[4,5]

SABAs can be administered through oral inhalation in multiple ways, including through metered-dose inhaler (MDI) with spacer, dry powder inhaler, and a nebulizer. In an MDI format, albuterol is 90 µg per puff or 2.5 mg/3 mL nebulizer ampoule. Smaller-dose nebulizer dosing is available at 1.25 mg/3 mL.[4] Salbutamol is 100 µg per puff and similarly 2.5 mg/3 mL nebulizer ampoule. Levalbuterol is 45 µg per puff and 1.25 µg/3 mL ampoule generally.[4] Dosing in an exacerbation is distributed by age. Global Initiative for Asthma (GINA) guideline recommendations for patients 5 years of age and younger are to use 2 puffs of SABA with a spacer up to every 3 to 4 hours. For patients 6 years of age and older, this can be increased to 4 to 8 puffs.[5] EPR-3 guidelines recommend up to 2 treatments spaced 20 minutes apart of 2 to 6 puffs of SABA through an MDI or nebulized treatment. The SABA treatment is then recommended every 3 to 4 hours for 24 to 48 hours.[4] This increase in SABA use is also generally accompanied by other increases in therapy described further in this article.

There are multiple side effects to consider with SABAs but the benefits far outweigh the potential side effects because of their effectiveness with bronchodilation. The most common side effects include tachycardia and tremors. Other possible side effects include headache, hypokalemia, and hyperglycemia. These side effects are more common when albuterol is dosed more frequently than every 4 hours, such as in the emergency room or during hospitalizations.[4]

A major drug interaction to consider for SABAs is β-blockers, which may decrease the efficacy of SABAs. Loop and thiazide diuretics may enhance the hypokalemic effect of beta agonists. Sympathomimetic drugs enhance tachycardia and tremors.[11]

Short-Acting Muscarinic Antagonist

Short-acting muscarinic antagonists (SAMAs) reverse cholinergically mediated bronchospasm.[4] SAMAs have been shown to have additive benefit to SABA when used in the emergency department.[4,12] If initiated at home in combination with SABA therapy, patients may benefit from the earlier initiation of the additive benefit. This treatment may prevent the need for further escalation of care.

SAMA dosing may vary by age.[4] According to the GINA guidelines, ipratropium bromide may be given at 2 puffs of 80 µg or 250 mg nebulized every 20 minutes for the first hour.[5] This dose is typically given in the emergency department. For ages 12 years and older, EPR-3 guidelines suggest 2 to 3 puffs of the 17 or 18 µg per puff MDI or 0.25 to 0.5 mg of a nebulized solution of ipratropium bromide every 6 hours with no specific recommendations made for those less than 12 years old.[4]

Common potential side effects to consider for SAMAs include drying of oral and respiratory secretions and blurred vision if sprayed in the eye. Bronchospasm is a rare side effect experienced by some individuals.[4] It is important to consider that SAMAs may enhance the effect of anticholinergic drugs and may decrease the effects of cholinergic drugs.[13]

SYSTEMIC ORAL CORTICOSTEROID

Oral steroids decrease airway inflammation in patients with asthma. Guidelines suggest consideration of oral steroids if the patient has an incomplete or poor response to SABA.[4] Steroids do not provide immediate benefit but may start to provide benefit within 3 hours of administration.[14] This point is important because patients with longer duration of symptoms are more likely to require hospital admission.[15] New pediatric evidence suggests that incorporation of a home supply of oral steroids into the home management of patients with moderate to severe asthma was associated with a significant decline in emergency department visits without any increase in hospitalizations or pediatric intensive care unit stays.[16]

Recommended dosage for oral corticosteroids in adults is 1 mg/kg/d, with a maximum dose of 50 to 60 mg for 5 to 7 days. Some patients require a longer course.[5,17] For children less than 12 years of age, the recommended dosage is 1 to 2 mg/kg/d for 3 to 5 days, with a maximum dose of 40 mg to 60 mg.[4,5,17] Pediatric patients may also require a longer course.[4]

Common side effects can include sleep disturbance, mood changes, psychosis, hypertension, and increased appetite.[5,17] When used for an extended period of time or very frequently, side effects may also include decreased bone mineral density, immunosuppression, adrenal suppression, delayed wound healing, cushingoid changes, and increase in psychiatric symptoms.[4,18] Despite an extensive list of potential side effects, the benefits of oral steroids outweigh the risks when treatment is required for the inflammation contributing to moderate to severe asthma exacerbations. Lack of appropriate treatment could result in severe morbidity and possible death.

Many drug-to-drug interactions exist with systemic corticosteroids. An all-inclusive list is beyond the scope of this article but common interactions include enhanced anticoagulation with warfarin, hypokalemia with loop diuretics, and enhanced adverse effects of NSAIDs. Systemic steroids diminish the effects of vaccinations. Of note, when given with cytochrome P3A4 (CYP3A4) inhibitors, the effects of corticosteroids are likely to increase as the serum concentration is increased.[19]

ADDITIONAL PHARMACOLOGIC INTERVENTIONS

In an attempt to decrease oral corticosteroid use and the associated extensive list of side effects, other options can be considered in the home management of an asthma exacerbation.

INHALED CORTICOSTEROID

Inhaled corticosteroids (ICSs) are a mainstay of long-term asthma controller therapy.[4] They work to decrease inflammation by inhibiting inflammatory cell migration and activation, which decreases airway hyperresponsiveness.[4] Intermittent use or increased doses of the controller therapy ICS can be used in the treatment of asthma exacerbations.[5] New evidence suggests that, in children less than 5 years of age with history of wheezing during respiratory infections, intermittent ICS use in conjunction with SABAs decreases risk of exacerbations requiring oral steroids compared with SABA use alone.[20–23] There was no difference in risk of exacerbation requiring oral steroids in a similar group when intermittent ICS dosing compared with ICS use as a controller.[24] In the limited number of studies done in patients aged 12 years and older, there was no significant difference in risk of exacerbation requiring oral steroids when comparing intermittent ICS with ICS controller versus ICS controller alone and intermittent ICS versus ICS controller.[25–28] A recent study in the United Kingdom showed that, in patients aged 16 years and older with asthma, quadrupling the dose of their ICS controllers resulted in fewer severe asthma exacerbations (based on use of systemic steroids or unscheduled health care visits) compared with the group that did not increase their

ICS dosing.[29] There was insufficient evidence to draw any conclusions for ages 5 to 11 years.[20]

GINA guidelines recommend increasing ICS dosing during an acute exacerbation to at least double the usual dosage, and possibly quadruple the normal dosage (a maximum of 2000 μg/d).[5] This dosage can be administered via MDI with spacer, dry powder inhaler, or nebulized solution.[4] ERP-3 specifically states that doubling the dose has not shown improved outcomes; however, this was associated with a study with delayed initiation of increased dosing.[5] These guidelines are being reevaluated in the context of the new evidence available regarding intermittent ICS use.[20]

Acute side effects of inhaled steroids include development of oral thrush, particularly if not using with a spacer and not rinsing the mouth after use. Other complaints include cough and dysphonia. Long term, there is a known effect on linear growth, although this seems to be dose dependent. At high doses there is the potential for adrenal suppression and development of Cushing syndrome along with the other aforementioned side effects of systemic corticosteroids.[4]

Several drug-drug interactions should be considered with ICS use. Fluticasone, budesonide, and mometasone specifically are metabolized by the CYP3A4 isoenzyme leading to interactions with drugs also metabolized by this system. Specifically, antifungal azole medications and ritonavir may increase concentrations of inhaled steroids.[4]

COMBINATION INHALED CORTICOSTEROID AND LONG-ACTING BETA AGONIST THERAPY

The long-acting beta agonist (LABA) formoterol has a fast onset of action similar to short-acting bronchodilators.[4,6] Studies in patients more than ages 12 years on maintenance combination therapy with ICS and formoterol have suggested that this combination can be used for symptom relief in acute exacerbations.[30] This treatment is often referred to as single maintenance and relief therapy (SMART) or adjustable maintenance dosing (AMD).[6,30]

There has been concern about the safety of SMART or AMD therapy in the United States because it is not approved by the US Food and Drug Administration (FDA).[6,31,32] It has been more readily adopted in Canada and European countries.[5,31] A systemic review and meta-analysis published in 2018 evaluated 16 trials of SMART. Fifteen of these trials evaluated budesonide and formoterol combination therapy. This meta-analysis showed decreased risk of asthma exacerbations requiring systemic oral steroids, hospitalization, or emergency department visit.[30] Supporters think that increasing the ICS dosing in combination with the long-acting beta agonist formoterol provides benefit from both therapies and allows ease of use with only 1 inhaler needed for both prevention and rescue treatment. Limited evidence exists for use in children between the ages of 4 and 11 years.[5,30,33,34] No evidence exists to support use in children less than 4 years of age.[30]

Various dosing of ICSs/LABAs were used in the studies reviewed. GINA guidelines suggest a maximum of 72 μg of formoterol in a day.[5] This dose can be administered via MDI with spacer or dry powder inhaler. However, this dose does exceed the FDA-approved dosing in the United States at this current time.[32]

Formoterol should only be used in combination with an ICS to avoid increased risk of asthma-related deaths.[4] Side effects and drug interactions of the ICS component were discussed earlier. Common potential side effects associated with formoterol include rhinitis, hypertension, tremors, and pharyngitis. Less common side effects include insomnia, hyperglycemia, hypokalemia, and tachycardia.[35] The likelihood of the less common side effects may increase with the higher dosing used in SMART. Potential side effects may be increased by drug-drug interactions. For example, formoterol may enhance tachycardia caused by short-acting bronchodilators and hypokalemia with loop diuretics. Caffeine may enhance the side effects and β-blockers may diminish the effect of formoterol.[35]

LONG-ACTING MUSCARINIC ANTAGONIST

Long-acting muscarinic antagonists (LAMAs) have become an important component in asthma care.[4,5] Tiotropium is the most common LAMA used in practice and in trials.[36] A recent systemic review and meta-analysis evaluated 15 trials that examined the effect of the addition of LAMA in asthma care. Only 2 trials evaluated children, including those aged 12 to 17 years. Compared with a placebo as add-on therapy to ICS, the LAMA therapy regimen showed an improvement in lung function in individual studies.[37–39] A meta-analysis of these studies showed a lower risk of asthma exacerbations requiring oral steroids.[36–39] There was no identified difference between the addition of a LAMA versus LABA. Combination of both LAMA and LABA with ICS did not show any additional decrease in asthma exacerbations but may improve spirometry and asthma symptom control scores.[20,36] The lack of rapid onset of the LAMA currently limits the potential for use for SMART and AMD.[20,40]

LAMA dosing may be adjusted by age and asthma severity.[40] Tiotropium 5 μg daily or 2.5 μg daily was used in trials for maintenance therapy.[36] This dose can be administered via a dry powder inhaler and a soft mist inhaler. Spacer use is not required with these forms.

Most common side effects to consider with LAMA therapy are pharyngitis, sinusitis, headache, and bronchitis.[40] Other adverse effects to consider include glaucoma, constipation, and dry mouth. Worsened bronchospasm is a rare side effect.[40] These side effects may be more prominent when LAMA is used in combination with other anticholinergic medications because of the potential for an additive effect.[40]

MACROLIDE THERAPY

There is limited evidence to support the use of macrolide therapy in acute asthma exacerbations, and routine use is not recommended in current asthma guidelines.[4–6,41] A study done in children aged 12 to 71 months with a history of recurrent severe wheezing suggested that azithromycin given at onset of viral symptoms prevented severe exacerbation of their respiratory symptoms.[42,43] A study focusing on children aged 1 to 3 years noted a decrease in symptom duration with exacerbation of respiratory symptoms after azithromycin administration.[44] This effect could not be duplicated in preschool-aged children prescribed azithromycin for wheezing after presentation to the emergency department.[45] In adults, azithromycin use in asthma exacerbations failed to show any benefit compared with placebo.[46] More research is needed on the topic of macrolides in asthma in all age ranges.

There is no standard dosing for oral/enteral azithromycin described in guidelines. Pediatric studies used 10 to 12 mg/kg/d.[4,5,41,42] A study done in the emergency department prescribed 10 mg/kg/d on the day of presentation followed by 5 mg/kg/d for 4 additional days.[45] In adults, the study described 500 mg daily for 3 days during an exacerbation.[46]

Side effects to consider with azithromycin therapy include hypersensitivity reactions, arrhythmias, vomiting, and diarrhea.[47] More data are required to evaluate the emergence of macrolide-resistant bacteria and alteration of the lung microbiome on macrolide therapy.[41]

Many potential drug interactions exist with azithromycin. It is important to recognize that macrolides may enhance the effects of QT interval–prolonging agents and the myopathic effects of some statin drugs. Macrolide therapy may also increase serum concentration of tacrolimus if used concurrently.[47]

LEUKOTRIENE RECEPTOR ANTAGONIST

Guidelines do not support routine use of intermittent leukotriene receptor antagonist (LTRA) therapy to treat asthma exacerbations. Studies on this treatment have had mixed results. One study did find modest benefit in reduction of symptoms and health care use when LTRA was used at the start of asthma symptoms in children aged 2 to 14 years with intermittent asthma.[48] A 2015 Cochrane Review found no evidence of benefit though when it was compared with a placebo in children aged 1 to 6 years who had history of episodic viral wheezing.[49] Studies in adults were also unable to show statistically significant benefit.[50,51] Further research is needed before a recommendation on intermittent LTRA use for asthma exacerbations can be made.

FUTURE CONSIDERATIONS/SUMMARY

Asthma is a common chronic disease in both adult and pediatric populations. Asthma exacerbations are common and proper management is essential to prevent mortality and decrease health care use. Many options exist to customize an asthma exacerbation management plan for patients at home. It is important to understand that it is not one size fits all with asthma management.

REFERENCES

1. Innes A. The global asthma Report 2018. Auckland (New Zealand): Global Asthma Network; 2018.
2. Centers for Disease Control. Twenty leading primary diagnosis groups and presence of chronic conditions at emergency department visits: United States. *Emergency Department Summary Tables.* 2015(Table 12). Available at: https://www.cdc.gov/nchs/data/nhamcs/web_tables/2015_ed_web_tables.pdf. Accessed January 9, 2019.
3. Centers for Disease Control. Most Recent Asthma Data. 2016. Available at: https://www.cdc.gov/asthma/most_recent_data.htm. Accessed January 19, 2019.
4. National Asthma Education and Prevention Program. Expert panel report 3 (EPR-3): guidelines for the diagnosis and management of asthma-summary report 2007. J Allergy Clin Immunol 2007;120(5 Suppl):S94–138.
5. Global Initiative for Asthma. Global Strategy for Asthma Management and Prevention. 2018. Available at: www.ginasthma.org. Accessed January 9,2019.
6. Dinakar C, Oppenheimer J, Portnoy J, et al. Management of acute loss of asthma control in the yellow zone: a practice parameter. Ann Allergy Asthma Immunol 2014;113(2):143–59.
7. Pinnock H, Parke HL, Panagioti M, et al. Systematic meta-review of supported self-management for asthma: a healthcare perspective. BMC Med 2017;15(1):64.
8. Leas BF, D'Anci KE, Apter AJ, et al. Effectiveness of indoor allergen reduction in asthma management: a systematic review. J Allergy Clin Immunol 2018;141(5):1854–69.
9. Wang Z, May SM, Charoenlap S, et al. Effects of secondhand smoke exposure on asthma morbidity and health care utilization in children: a systematic review and meta-analysis. Ann Allergy Asthma Immunol 2015;115(5):396–401.e2.

10. Bayly JE, Bernat D, Porter L, et al. Secondhand exposure to aerosols from electronic nicotine delivery systems and asthma exacerbations among youth with asthma. Chest 2019;155(1):88–93.
11. Albuterol. Lexi-Drugs. Lexicomp Online. Wolters Kluwer Health, Inc. Available at: http://online.lexi.com/lco/action/doc/retrieve/docid/patch_f/6292. Accessed January 21, 2019.
12. Aaron SD. The use of ipratropium bromide for the management of acute asthma exacerbation in adults and children: a systematic review. J Asthma 2001;38(7): 521–30.
13. Ipratropium (Oral Inhalation. Lexi-Drugs. Lexicomp Online. Wolters Kluwer Health, Inc. Available at: http://online.lexi.com/lco/action/doc/retrieve/docid/patch_f/1797824#rfs. Accessed January 21, 2019.
14. Rubin BK, Marcushamer S, Priel I, et al. Emergency management of the child with asthma. Pediatr Pulmonol 1990;8(1):45–57.
15. Kelly AM, Powell C, Kerr D. Patients with a longer duration of symptoms of acute asthma are more likely to require admission to hospital. Emerg Med (Fremantle) 2002;14(2):142–5.
16. Sarzynski LM, Turner T, Stukus DR, et al. Home supply of emergency oral steroids and reduction in asthma healthcare utilization. Pediatr Pulmonol 2017;52(12): 1546–9.
17. Fergeson JE, Patel SS, Lockey RF. Acute asthma, prognosis, and treatment. J Allergy Clin Immunol 2017;139(2):438–47.
18. Wang E, Hoyte FC. Traditional therapies for severe asthma. Immunol Allergy Clin North Am 2016;36(3):581–608.
19. Prednisone. Lexi-Drugs. Lexicomp Online. Wolters Kluwer Health, Inc. Available at: http://online.lexi.com/lco/action/doc/retrieve/docid/chibus_f/217959. Accessed January 21, 2019.
20. Sobieraj DM, Baker WL, Weeda ER, et al. Intermittent inhaled corticosteroids and long-acting muscarinic antagonists for asthma. Comparative effectiveness review No. 194. (Prepared by the University of Connecticut Evidence-based Practice Center under Contract No. 290-2015- 00012-I.) AHRQ Publication No. 17(18)-EHC027-EF. Rockville (MD): Agency for Healthcare Research and Quality; 2018.
21. Bacharier LB, Phillips BR, Zeiger RS, et al. Episodic use of an inhaled corticosteroid or leukotriene receptor antagonist in preschool children with moderate-to-severe intermittent wheezing. J Allergy Clin Immunol 2008;122(6):1127–35.e8.
22. Ducharme FM, Lemire C, Noya FJ, et al. Preemptive use of high-dose fluticasone for virus-induced wheezing in young children. N Engl J Med 2009;360(4):339–53.
23. Svedmyr J, Nyberg E, Thunqvist P, et al. Prophylactic intermittent treatment with inhaled corticosteroids of asthma exacerbations due to airway infections in toddlers. Acta Paediatr 1999;88(1):42–7.
24. Zeiger RS, Mauger D, Bacharier LB, et al. Daily or intermittent budesonide in preschool children with recurrent wheezing. N Engl J Med 2011;365(21):1990–2001.
25. Boushey HA, Sorkness CA, King TS, et al. Daily versus as-needed corticosteroids for mild persistent asthma. N Engl J Med 2005;352(15):1519–28.
26. Harrison TW, Oborne J, Newton S, et al. Doubling the dose of inhaled corticosteroid to prevent asthma exacerbations: randomised controlled trial. Lancet 2004; 363(9405):271–5.
27. Lahdensuo A, Haahtela T, Herrala J, et al. Randomised comparison of guided self management and traditional treatment of asthma over one year. BMJ 1996; 312(7033):748–52.

28. Oborne J, Mortimer K, Hubbard RB, et al. Quadrupling the dose of inhaled corticosteroid to prevent asthma exacerbations: a randomized, double-blind, placebo-controlled, parallel-group clinical trial. Am J Respir Crit Care Med 2009; 180(7):598–602.

29. McKeever T, Mortimer K, Wilson A, et al. Quadrupling inhaled glucocorticoid dose to abort asthma exacerbations. N Engl J Med 2018;378(10):902–10.

30. Sobieraj DM, Weeda ER, Nguyen E, et al. Association of inhaled corticosteroids and long-acting beta-agonists as controller and quick relief therapy with exacerbations and symptom control in persistent asthma: a systematic review and meta-analysis. JAMA 2018;319(14):1485–96.

31. FitzGerald JM, Sears MR, Boulet LP, et al. Adjustable maintenance dosing with budesonide/formoterol reduces asthma exacerbations compared with traditional fixed dosing: a five-month multicentre Canadian study. Can Respir J 2003;10(8): 427–34.

32. Polk BI, Dinakar C. Management of acute loss of asthma control: yellow zone strategies. Curr Opin Allergy Clin Immunol 2019;19(2):154–60.

33. Bisgaard H, Le Roux P, Bjamer D, et al. Budesonide/formoterol maintenance plus reliever therapy: a new strategy in pediatric asthma. Chest 2006;130(6):1733–43.

34. Papi A, Corradi M, Pigeon-Francisco C, et al. Beclometasone-formoterol as maintenance and reliever treatment in patients with asthma: a double-blind, randomised controlled trial. Lancet Respir Med 2013;1(1):23–31.

35. Formoterol. Lexi-Drugs. Lexicomp Online. Wolters Kluwer Health, Inc. Available at: http://online.lexi.com/lco/action/doc/retrieve/docid/pdh_f/130111. Accessed January 21, 2019.

36. Sobieraj DM, Baker WL, Nguyen E, et al. Association of inhaled corticosteroids and long-acting muscarinic antagonists with asthma control in patients with uncontrolled, persistent asthma: a systematic review and meta-analysis. JAMA 2018;319(14):1473–84.

37. Hamelmann E, Bateman ED, Vogelberg C, et al. Tiotropium add-on therapy in adolescents with moderate asthma: A 1-year randomized controlled trial. J Allergy Clin Immunol 2016;138(2):441–50.e8.

38. Ohta K, Ichinose M, Tohda Y, et al. Long-term once-daily tiotropium respimat(R) is well tolerated and maintains efficacy over 52 weeks in patients with symptomatic asthma in japan: a randomised, placebo-controlled study. PLoS One 2015;10(4): e0124109.

39. Paggiaro P, Halpin DM, Buhl R, et al. The effect of tiotropium in symptomatic asthma despite low- to medium-dose inhaled corticosteroids: a randomized controlled trial. J Allergy Clin Immunol Pract 2016;4(1):104–13.e2.

40. Spiriva® Respimat® (tiotropium bromide) inhalation spray [package insert]. Ridgefield (CT): Boehringer Ingelheim Pharmaceuticals, Inc; 2018.

41. Wong EH, Porter JD, Edwards MR, et al. The role of macrolides in asthma: current evidence and future directions. Lancet Respir Med 2014;2(8):657–70.

42. Raissy HH, Blake K. Macrolides for acute wheezing episodes in preschool children. Pediatr Allergy Immunol Pulmonol 2016;29(2):100–3.

43. Bacharier LB, Guilbert TW, Mauger DT, et al. Early administration of azithromycin and prevention of severe lower respiratory tract illnesses in preschool children with a history of such illnesses: a randomized clinical trial. JAMA 2015;314(19): 2034–44.

44. Stokholm J, Chawes BL, Vissing NH, et al. Azithromycin for episodes with asthma-like symptoms in young children aged 1-3 years: a randomised, double-blind, placebo-controlled trial. Lancet Respir Med 2016;4(1):19–26.

45. Mandhane PJ, Paredes Zambrano de Silbernagel P, Aung YN, et al. Treatment of preschool children presenting to the emergency department with wheeze with azithromycin: a placebo-controlled randomized trial. PLoS One 2017;12(8): e0182411.
46. Johnston SL, Szigeti M, Cross M, et al. Azithromycin for acute exacerbations of asthma : The AZALEA randomized clinical trial. JAMA Intern Med 2016;176(11): 1630–7.
47. Azithromycin. Lexi-Drugs. Lexicomp Online. Wolters Kluwer Health, Inc. Available at: http://online.lexi.com/lco/action/doc/retrieve/docid/patch_f/1768824. Accessed January 21, 2019.
48. Robertson CF, Price D, Henry R, et al. Short-course montelukast for intermittent asthma in children: a randomized controlled trial. Am J Respir Crit Care Med 2007;175(4):323–9.
49. Brodlie M, Gupta A, Rodriguez-Martinez CE, et al. Leukotriene receptor antagonists as maintenance and intermittent therapy for episodic viral wheeze in children. Cochrane Database Syst Rev 2015;(10):CD008202.
50. Watts K, Chavasse RJ. Leukotriene receptor antagonists in addition to usual care for acute asthma in adults and children. Cochrane Database Syst Rev 2012;(5):CD006100.
51. Zubairi AB, Salahuddin N, Khawaja A, et al. A randomized, double-blind, placebo-controlled trial of oral montelukast in acute asthma exacerbation. BMC Pulm Med 2013;13:20.

How Dr Google Is Impacting Parental Medical Decision Making

David R. Stukus, MD

KEYWORDS

• Internet • Evidence-based information • Social media • Self-management

KEY POINTS

- The use of online search engines to find health-related information is commonplace.
- Non-evidence-based Web sites include misinformation and advice regarding unproven alternative therapies, pseudoscientific explanations, and personal anecdotes.
- Medical professionals need to have awareness of misconceptions that interfere with parental medical decision making and be prepared to actively discuss this during clinical encounters.

INTRODUCTION

The patient-provider relationship is sacred. Patients trust their physicians with intimate details surrounding their health and relay concerns they may not even be comfortable discussing with their spouse. In return, physicians protect their patient's privacy and offer information and advice to help them achieve optimal health outcomes. Shared medical decision making relies on trust from both ends of this relationship. However, what happens when patients go outside this relationship to obtain information pertaining to their own care, or that of their children? What happens when patients or parents feel their physician is not listening to their concerns or offering options that are incompatible with their personal belief systems? Patients cannot be faulted for searching for medical information online. After all, we live in a world connected in real time and society functions through use of the Internet, social media, and constant access to handheld devices. However, when the information patients seek turns out to be incorrect, or even harmful, this can not only damage the patient-provider relationship but also lead patients to seek non-evidence-based promises of miracle cures, costly treatments, or unnecessary testing. If physicians and medical professionals are to continue to help patients and parents achieve the best health outcomes, then they will need to

Disclosure Statement: Consultant for Aimmune and Before Brands, Inc.

Division of Allergy and Immunology, Nationwide Children's Hospital, The Ohio State University College of Medicine, 700 Children's Drive, Columbus, OH 43205, USA

E-mail address: David.stukus@nationwidechildrens.org

Immunol Allergy Clin N Am 39 (2019) 583–591
https://doi.org/10.1016/j.iac.2019.07.011   immunology.theclinics.com

evolve. This evolution begins by appreciating the various types of misinformation that impacts medical decision making and developing approaches to address this during individual clinical encounters.

DR GOOGLE WILL SEE YOU NOW

There are many reasons patients or parents may seek medical information online, starting with easy, immediate access to information 24 hours a day, 7 days a week and at their convenience. It is simply much easier to type in a few key words on a search engine than try to call a physician's office, leave a message, and wait for a reply. Well-child visits with a pediatrician typically take place every few months during the first 2 years of life, but then generally occur only once a year thereafter. During the months between visits, children will exhibit a range of normal developmental changes, childhood illnesses, and other symptoms that may raise concern from parents. Rashes, stomach pains, changes to bowel habits, sleep disruptions, behavioral changes, and upper respiratory infections are all normal expected parts of childhood but are also common sources of parental concern. A visit to the pediatrician may provide reassurance, but this necessitates time off work and school, copayments, and travel. It is simply much easier for parents to take their questions online through search engines or social media groups.

Problems arise when parents type their queries into search engines such as Google. These search engines use various algorithms to display results with the top search items often reflecting the most popular sites, or those that have paid to appear at the top of the list. It is natural to assume that the sites that appear at the top of a page are the most important and even the most accurate. Unfortunately, this is rarely the case. There is no regulation of any Web sites in regards to vetting the medical information they provide, a concept that many people may not understand. People commonly assume that prominent physicians such as Mehmet Oz, also known as Dr Oz, are trustworthy and that their advice is accurate and evidence based. After all, why would a major television network give Dr Oz a syndicated talk show unless he was trustworthy? Unfortunately, non-evidence-based approaches and alternative medicine products are frequently discussed and promoted through the Dr Oz show, which has led to congressional hearings and discussion from policymakers regarding the need for more accountability.[1]

All medical professionals should spend time perusing the Internet to acquaint themselves with the information, and more importantly, misinformation that their patients are encountering online. It can be as easy as typing common questions encountered in the clinical setting into a search engine and then going through the sites that appear. It is known that two-thirds of adults will search for health-related information online and not just for themselves but also for friends or family members as well.[2] The information they discover will influence how they perceive their own health and may lead to inaccurate self-diagnosis, use of non-evidence-based and costly at-home testing kits, inappropriate expectations regarding treatment outcomes, and ultimately, dissatisfaction with the care they receive from "traditional" Western medicine. If medical professionals can better understand where their patients are coming from in regards to this type of information, they can address this during clinical encounters and offer anticipatory guidance as well as words of caution regarding online searches. Lastly, medical professionals should also be familiar with the evidence surrounding the same types of searches, including what is available through peer-reviewed published research and clinical guidelines. There is often a large discrepancy between information found on Google compared with PubMed. For instance, at the time of this writing, a search for the term "artificial red dye allergy" in Google yields 5.1 million results, whereas the same search in PubMed yields 3 results, none of which are relevant or actually demonstrate that this is a proven (or plausible) diagnosis.

MISCONCEPTIONS SURROUNDING ALLERGIC CONDITIONS

Allergic conditions are particularly susceptible to misinformation, pseudoscience, nonvalidated testing, and anecdotes describing success rates from treatment that far surpasses anything reported in peer-reviewed literature. Atopic dermatitis, asthma, allergic rhinitis, food allergy, and drug allergy are all very common conditions that impact millions of people. Children are particularly susceptible, and parents can easily become frustrated owing to a lack of any current cure for their child with atopic dermatitis, asthma, or food allergies. These conditions are known to have significant psychosocial consequences, including poor sleep, missed school (or work for parents), and behavioral changes, and can lead to bullying.[3] In addition, food allergies can be potentially life threatening, and the number one fear expressed by parents of children with peanut allergy is that their child may die from accidental exposure, including from trace amounts.[4] Because of the highly emotional nature of these concerns, these parents are particularly susceptible to seeking alternative approaches and spending money, time, and emotional investments on nonvalidated testing or treatment options.

Patient or parent testimonials touting the benefits of non-evidence-based treatment approaches are rampant on Web sites, and particularly on social media. Medical professionals are well versed in the important differences between anecdotes and evidence, but the lay public often equates the two. Anecdotes can provide powerful and emotional stories that relay tales of miracle cures or improvement through various means. These personal stories do not serve as evidence and may have no applicability to anyone else's health. First, there is no proof that these stories are true or actually happened. Even if true, anecdotes are highly subject to multiple forms of bias, and important pertinent details are often neglected or ignored. Almost all chronic medical conditions exhibit a normal pattern of waxing and waning symptoms, which is frustrating for parents and patients. This also allows for misattributing association with causality. For instance, if someone with atopic dermatitis exhibits a flare of symptoms during the winter months or while acutely ill and decides to eliminate gluten from their diet at the same time, they can easily misattribute their gluten avoidance as the "treatment" when their skin ultimately improves. Should they choose to share their story online or with the social media followers, then others will inappropriately encounter advice on how a gluten-free diet can treat atopic dermatitis.

Table 1 lists a few examples of nonvalidated tests or treatment options found online that pertain to common allergic conditions. These examples are constantly changing, often matching whatever new fad or celebrity testimonial is currently en vogue. Given

Table 1	
Examples of nonvalidated testing and treatment options found online	
Diagnostic Testing	**Treatment Options**
Immunoglobulin G tests for food allergy or sensitivity	Chiropractic adjustments
Provocation-neutralization	Himalayan salt therapy for asthma
Applied kinesiology	Nambudripad's allergy elimination technique
Cytotoxic testing	Lifestyle eating and performance
Electrodermal analysis	
Chemical analysis of hair and urine	

their public profile, actors, actresses, and musicians often have very large platforms and can reach millions of people from across the world. Regardless of the fact that most celebrities lack any education, training, or experience that would give them any qualifications whatsoever to dispense medical advice, this has not prevented many celebrities from influencing the medical decision making of their fans. Actress Gwyneth Paltrow founded a company, Goop, that promotes various forms of wellness and medical advice targeting women. Subscribers encounter non-evidence-based advice touting the benefits of cleanses for weight loss, jade eggs for improved sexual performance, and bee venom for treatment of wrinkles. Another actress and former Playboy model, Jenny McCarthy, has used her popularity to actively promote the harms of childhood vaccines and used the personal story of her son's autism to reinforce the common misconception (despite sound evidence to the contrary) that vaccines cause autism. The President of the United States, Donald Trump, has also publicly declared vaccines to be harmful and has even stated that physicians are engaging in a conspiracy to harm their patients. Due in part to these endorsements, the antivaccine movement has gained significant traction across the world and has led to recent measles outbreaks in multiple countries, including the United States, a country in which measles was officially eradicated in 2000.[5] In early 2019, the World Health Organization listed vaccine hesitancy as one of the top 10 threats to global health.[6] Needless to say, celebrities and politicians who publicly dispense incorrect medical advice absolutely impact the decision making of patients.

LOW HEALTH LITERACY

Health literacy refers to the capacity of someone to understand, interpret, and apply medical information to self-management skills. This is more than just the ability to read. Health literacy encompasses the ability to make effective decisions pertaining to one's own medical care. Only 12% of adults in the United States are deemed to have proficient health literacy.[7] Patients with low health literacy are less likely to receive annual influenza vaccines, schedule and appear for routine medical appointments, and take medication as directed by their prescription.[8] All together, this contributes to suboptimal health outcomes and increased risk for hospitalization.

There are validated instruments available to determine each patient's or parent's level of health literacy. However, use of these questionnaires is time consuming and can disrupt clinic flow, which makes them challenging to implement in routine clinical practice. Even if formal instruments are not used, medical providers can still improve their understanding of health literacy and address this with patients during each visit. Elderly patients and those who speak English as a second language are at increased risk to have low health literacy.[9] However, any patient who has difficulty filling out questionnaires pertaining to their medical history, who cannot accurately recount their medication prescriptions, or who appears to be confused when discussing medical information warrants additional attention. With heightened awareness, medical professionals can actively monitor for warning signs of low health literacy and address this during the visit.

The concepts surrounding low health literacy are important given its prevalence and also how it can impact patient and parental decision making pertaining to the information they encounter online. People with low health literacy are more susceptible to the common misinformation tactics found through online searches for medical information. They will be less likely to recognize deliberate misinformation from those selling products and more susceptible to fanciful claims and pseudoscientific explanations. If medical professionals can improve their own recognition of low health literacy among their patients, then they can actively address this when discussing treatment recommendations or issues pertaining to self-management. There are simple tools that can be used to improve retention of important medical information after the visit. The Ask-Me-3 questions[10] encompass 3 questions that assess a patient's understanding of their self-management plan:

1. What is my main problem?
2. What do I need to do (about the problem)?
3. Why is it important for me to do this?

It would be remarkable if every patient could answer these simple questions at the conclusion of each medical visit. Another method called the Teachback Method relies on the patient to reiterate the medical information given to them during their visit. By using the Teachback Method, medical professionals are forced to prioritize the information they give, keep the information simple, and make it pertinent. Then, if the patient cannot accurately reiterate the information they are given, the onus is on the provider to take another approach or use a different explanation. This ensures that the person doing the educating meets the learner where they are at in regards to their level of understanding and ability to understand. For example, an allergist may wish to educate a parent of a newly diagnosed asthmatic child with all the information pertaining to the immunopathology surrounding their asthma, association with other atopic conditions, and range of available treatment options. However, the message the parent may most benefit from at this visit is likely much more simple, along the lines of: "Your child has asthma, which causes his airways to be irritated and have recurrent episodes of tightening. Albuterol is a medicine that works very quickly to reverse that tightening when it occurs and should be used as soon as he has persistent cough, difficulty breathing, or wakes at night due to cough. The way we give albuterol is very important, so we're going to review the proper technique and practice with you today."

LOW SCIENCE LITERACY

The ability to trust and understand science is another area where celebrities and policymakers influence the opinions of the general public. Frustration often mounts from patients and the general public because of the ever-changing evidence and clinical guidelines. As evidence accumulates, it often changes the understanding of underlying disease pathogenesis, prognosis, and best approaches to treatment. An example pertaining to pediatric allergy pertains to advice surrounding the timing of introduction of allergenic foods, particularly peanut. In 2000, the American Academy of Pediatrics (AAP) recommended avoiding cow's milk until 1 year of age, egg until 2 years of age, and peanut, tree nuts, and seafood until 3 years of age.[11] This recommendation was based on expert opinion and the understanding at the time that avoiding exposure may prevent the development of food allergy. Within just 8 years, the AAP removed that advice and offered a general recommendation that those foods do not need to be avoided, but did not include an active recommendation to introduce these foods. In 2015, the Learning Early About Peanut study demonstrated for the first time that early introduction of peanut into the diet of infants at risk to develop peanut allergy (moderate to severe eczema and/or egg allergy) before 12 months of age AND ongoing ingestion at least 3 times a week up to the age of 5 years old dramatically reduced the development of peanut allergy compared with infants who avoided any peanut ingestion.[12] This prompted the publication of new guidelines in 2017 that recommend active introduction of age-appropriate peanut products to all infants around 4 to 6 months of age, followed by ongoing ingestion, with risk stratification and provisions for peanut immunoglobulin E testing before introduction for infants with moderate to severe eczema and/or egg allergy.[13] Ultimately, within 17 years, the recommendations surrounding the timing and manner of introducing peanut into an infant's diet changed dramatically. Allergists and medical professionals view this as an excellent example of scientific achievement and progress. This is how science and clinical guidelines should evolve; this is proof that the system is working. However, parents and those with low science literacy may view this as another reason to distrust science and even physicians. After all, if we cannot make up our mind about something like when to feed babies peanut, then how can they trust anything else we have to say?

In addition, distrust of evidence leads to climate change denialism, vaccine hesitancy, belief that genetically modified organisms are unhealthy, and even that the Earth is flat. It is important for medical professionals to be aware of low science literacy because this will be present among the patients and parents who come to the office every day. A researcher poses a question and systematically attempts to identify evidence that answers that question, giving equal weight to evidence in support of and against the hypothesis. However, many online searches, particularly by those with low science literacy, start with someone thinking they know the answer (or mistaking their opinion as fact) and then seeking Web sites or resources that reinforce their already formulated beliefs. This is confirmation bias and another contributing factor that influences how parents make medical decisions pertaining to their child's care.

MEDIA HEADLINES

Health-related topics often generate interest, and media outlets are constantly searching for the latest publications or presentations at national meetings. Unfortunately, the headlines are often inaccurate, and copyright editors choose phrasing that is more likely to generate Web site clicks and shares and less likely to be scientifically accurate. It is impossible to accurately describe the nuances of a peer-reviewed study, such as inclusion/exclusion criteria, methodology, results, limitations, and findings in 1 headline, yet people often use the headlines alone and never even read the article (which often misconstrues the research as well). An astonishing 59% of links shared on Twitter are never even read by the person sharing them with others.[14] Thus, media reports and catchy headlines that misinterpret, overstate, or confuse research findings can be easily misinterpreted. Medical professionals can set a Google alert for articles related to any topic of interest and receive a current and updated array of examples, which can be valuable for addressing with patients. In addition, medical professionals should take the time to identify recent popular medical headlines, *then* read the article, and *then* locate and read the actual research study. More often than not, the information provided in the article is either missing the mark in regards to overall study findings or cherry picked 1 particular aspect that was deemed more popular or likely to generate interest while ignoring important study limitations or additional findings. This approach can offer valuable insight into how parents formulate their own medical decisions.

COGNITIVE BIAS

Everyone has cognitive biases, which are systematic patterns that deviate from the norm and interfere with their ability to make rational decisions. Health care professionals who have a thorough understanding of cognitive biases and how they can dramatically impact one's perception of reality will easily recognize these during patient encounters and throughout online searches. This can help not only better understand online behavior but also offer a unique advantage during personal interactions. If medical professionals can understand and identify the common faults in how people make decisions related to their health, they can point these out, provide a rational explanation, and ideally assist medical decision making.

Cognitive biases lead people to create their own personal subjective reality, which can dictate behavior. As one can imagine, if everyone is viewing the world according to their own perception, this can lead to false conclusions that lie well outside proven facts, science, and reality. It behooves health care professionals to appreciate the wide range of viewpoints, biases, and alternate perceptions of reality that are disseminated online and particularly how this can influence parental attitudes and decision making.

PSEUDOSCIENCE 101

The boundary between science and pseudoscience is often murky. Pseudoscience essentially consists of statements, beliefs, or practices that are claimed to be both scientific and factual, but are incompatible with the scientific method. Online searches for medical information offer a perfect platform for attention-grabbing headlines and pseudoscientific explanations for unproven diagnostic testing or treatment options to gain traction and widespread appeal. Those headlines that claim black mold causes hidden toxicity, the benefits of detoxes and cleanses, or how gluten causes leaky-gut syndrome: those are pseudoscience 101. Why does the public fall for this, often to the point of spending large amounts of money for treatment options or programs that are not supported by any evidence? Cognitive biases contribute, but another phenomenon may be contributing to this as well and is rooted in poor communication skills by medical professionals.

Traditionally, science has been communicated to the public by those in academics, who, to the average person, may seem elitist, nerdy, or disconnected. However, scientists and health care professionals have generally missed the mark when trying to communicate health-related information to the general public. It is known that people are searching online for health-related information. As such, this space has been filled by professionals who overreach their qualifications, such as chiropractors, homeopaths, naturopaths, and other alternative medicine providers (plus the occasional board-certified physician who has crossed over to the dark side of pedaling pseudoscience in the name of profit). These individuals have traditionally excelled at communicating and listening to patients, which, in turn, makes them seem more trustworthy and believable. Although some of these individuals deliberately dispense misinformation in an attempt to profit from their services, many are subject to the Dunning-Kruger effect and are merely explaining things in a way they were actually taught in their alternative medicine education. They simply do not know what they do not know and fill in the gaps with thought processes that are often not physiologically plausible and rarely supported by evidence. Regardless of intent, this is an important arena that contributes to the vast array of misinformation online, confuses patients and the public, and by muddying the waters, ultimately leads to decreased trust in qualified health care professionals who are dispensing evidence-based information.

Unfortunately, modern medicine has failed to find a cure, and in some cases effective treatment, for many chronic conditions. Patients can easily become frustrated when health care professionals dismiss their chronic ailments and concerns or fail to provide any relief. It is only natural for them to turn to unproven therapies in the quest to find relief from their struggles. This is where they can be taken advantage of through promises of magical cures or providers who claim to know the "cause" of their complaints (occasionally with disparaging remarks about how medical schools do not teach the "right" information). Chronic Lyme disease, chelation therapy, vaccine toxicity, toxic mold syndrome, electromagnetic sensitivity, and bogus cancer treatments are just a few areas where pseudoscience prevails. Harm occurs when patients forego proven evidence-based treatment options in favor of unproven therapies, spend significant amounts of money, and experience side effects, at times severe, from pursuing this path. This is one of the most profound reasons health care professionals should disseminate evidence-based information through social media: to try to reach some of these patients and prevent their descent into the realm of pseudoscience.

Use of specific wording, conspiracy-fueled rejection of evidence-based recommendations, and cherry-picked data from research studies performed in laboratory animals or presented as abstracts at scientific meetings but not published in peer-reviewed journals are a few tactics used by those peddling pseudoscience. Health care professionals can assist patients and the public in identifying and avoiding pseudoscience by promoting positive messaging on social media and raising awareness.

HOW MEDICAL PROFESSIONALS CAN REGAIN TRUST

By recognizing that patients and parents are going online to search for health information, medical professionals can actively discuss this at each clinical encounter. This should be actively discussed in a nonthreatening manner and offer acknowledgment that this occurs. Providers should allow for questions to be raised, even if they stem from areas that are far outside the plausible realm, and appreciate that most patients *want* to hear proper evidence-based information to assist their medical decision making.

Medical providers can use this example phrasing as an opening to this discussion: "I realize you have likely spent some time searching for information online. There are many great resources available that offer evidence-based information. Unfortunately, there are also many non-evidenced sources that provide incorrect, and possibly harmful, information. Please feel free to ask me any questions about the information you have read, particularly if it differs significantly from the information I provide to you. If you'd like, I am happy to provide you with a list of trusted resources that provide vetted information. I do recommend caution if you encounter personal stories or information surrounding treatment that sounds too good to be true, as that is often the case."

Although all of this can serve as a source of frustration for medical professionals, it is important to embrace how the world has become so interactive and the multiple benefits that online resources provide. Providers who fail to adapt may be seen as old fashioned or less trustworthy by patients. As society evolves, the millennial generation will get older and start to have children of their own. It behooves providers to interact with these individuals in a manner to which they are accustomed. Although mid to older generations of physicians and medical providers may recall growing up in a world with rotary telephones, they must appreciate that younger generations have only known an online world. If the valued patient-provider relationship is to be resurrected, then providers must evolve as well.

SUMMARY

Now more than ever, it is important for medical professionals to appreciate the sheer amount of health information available online. It is even more important to appreciate the sheer amount of misinformation available as well. By actively spending time online searching for information from the patient perspective, providers will gain a new understanding of where their patients and parents of their patients are coming from. This knowledge can then translate to individual conversations in the clinical setting and can assist decision making.

REFERENCES

1. Tilburt JC, Allyse M, Hafferty FW. The case of Dr. Oz: ethics, evidence, and does professional self-regulation work? AMA J Ethics 2017;19(2):199–206.
2. Lawhon L. New survey reveals importance of online health communities. Philadelphia: Health Union, LLC; 2016. Available at: health-union.com/news/online-health-experience-survey/.
3. Herbert L, Shemesh E, Bender B. Clinical management of psychosocial concerns related to food allergy. J Allergy Clin Immunol Pract 2016;4(2):205–13.
4. DunnGalvin A, Dubois AE, Flokstra-de Blok BM, et al. The effects of food allergy on quality of life. Chem Immunol Allergy 2015;101:235–52.
5. Olive JK, Hotez PJ, Damania A, et al. Correction: the state of the antivaccine movement in the United States: a focused examination of nonmedical exemptions in states and counties. PLoS Med 2018;15(7):e1002616.
6. Ten threats to global health in 2019. Available at: https://www.who.int/emergencies/ten-threats-to-global-health-in-2019. Accessed March 15, 2019.
7. Kirsch IS, Jungeblut A, Jenkins L, et al. Adult literacy in America: a first look at the results of the national adult literacy survey (NALS). Washington, DC: National Center for Education Statistics, U.S. Department of Education; 1993.
8. Scott TL, Gazmararian JA, Williams MV, et al. Health literacy and preventive health care use among Medicare enrollees in a managed care organization. Med Care 2002;40(5):395–404.
9. National Center for Education Statistics. The health literacy of America's adults: results from the 2003 national assessment of adult literacy. Washington, DC: U.S. Department of Education; 2006.
10. Michalopoulou G, Falzarano P, Arfken C, et al. Implementing Ask Me 3 to improve African American patient satisfaction and perceptions of physician cultural competency. J Cult Divers 2010;17(2):62–7.
11. Kleinman RE. American Academy of Pediatrics recommendations for complementary feeding. Pediatrics 2000;106(Suppl 4):1274.
12. Du Toit G, Roberts G, Sayre PH, et al. Randomized trial of peanut consumption in infants at risk for peanut allergy. N Engl J Med 2015;372(9):803–13.
13. Togias A, Cooper SF, Acebal ML, et al. Addendum guidelines for the prevention of peanut allergy in the United States: report of the National Institute of Allergy and Infectious Diseases-sponsored expert panel. J Allergy Clin Immunol 2017; 139(1):29–44.
14. Gabielkov M, Ramachandran A, Chaintreau A, et al. Social clicks: what and who gets read on twitter? ACM SIGMETRICS/IFIP performance 2016, HAL archives. Jun 2016 2016. Antibes Juan-les-Pins, (France).

UNITED STATES POSTAL SERVICE® Statement of Ownership, Management, and Circulation (All Periodicals Publications Except Requester Publications)

1. Publication Title	2. Publication Number	3. Filing Date
IMMUNOLOGY AND ALLERGY CLINICS OF NORTH AMERICA	006 – 361	9/18/2019

4. Issue Frequency	5. Number of Issues Published Annually	6. Annual Subscription Price
FEB, MAY, AUG, NOV	4	$341.00

7. Complete Mailing Address of Known Office of Publication (Not printer) (Street, city, county, state, and ZIP+4®)

ELSEVIER INC.
230 Park Avenue, Suite 800
New York, NY 10169

Contact Person
STEPHEN R. BUSHING

Telephone (Include area code)
215-239-3688

8. Complete Mailing Address of Headquarters or General Business Office of Publisher (Not printer)

ELSEVIER INC.
230 Park Avenue, Suite 800
New York, NY 10169

9. Full Names and Complete Mailing Addresses of Publisher, Editor, and Managing Editor (Do not leave blank)

Publisher (Name and complete mailing address)

TAYLOR BALL, ELSEVIER INC.
1600 JOHN F KENNEDY BLVD. SUITE 1800
PHILADELPHIA, PA 19103-2899

Editor (Name and complete mailing address)

KATERINA HEIDHAUSEN, ELSEVIER INC.
1600 JOHN F KENNEDY BLVD. SUITE 1800
PHILADELPHIA, PA 19103-2899

Managing Editor (Name and complete mailing address)

PATRICK MANLEY, ELSEVIER INC.
1600 JOHN F KENNEDY BLVD. SUITE 1800
PHILADELPHIA, PA 19103-2899

10. Owner (Do not leave blank. If the publication is owned by a corporation, give the name and address of the corporation immediately followed by the names and addresses of all stockholders owning or holding 1 percent or more of the total amount of stock. If not owned by a corporation, give the names and addresses of the individual owners. If owned by a partnership or other unincorporated firm, give its name and address as well as those of each individual owner. If the publication is published by a nonprofit organization, give its name and address.)

Full Name	Complete Mailing Address
WHOLLY OWNED SUBSIDIARY OF REED/ELSEVIER, US HOLDINGS	1600 JOHN F KENNEDY BLVD. SUITE 1800 PHILADELPHIA, PA 19103-2899

11. Known Bondholders, Mortgagees, and Other Security Holders Owning or Holding 1 Percent or More of Total Amount of Bonds, Mortgages, or Other Securities. If none, check box ▸ ☐ None

Full Name	Complete Mailing Address
N/A	

12. Tax Status (For completion by nonprofit organizations authorized to mail at nonprofit rates) (Check one)
The purpose, function, and nonprofit status of this organization and the exempt status for federal income tax purposes:
☒ Has Not Changed During Preceding 12 Months
☐ Has Changed During Preceding 12 Months (Publisher must submit explanation of change with this statement)

PS Form **3526**, July 2014 (Page 1 of 4 (see instructions page 4)) PSN: 7530-01-000-9931 PRIVACY NOTICE: See our privacy policy on www.usps.com.

---

13. Publication Title	14. Issue Date for Circulation Data Below
IMMUNOLOGY AND ALLERGY CLINICS OF NORTH AMERICA	MAY 2019

15. Extent and Nature of Circulation			Average No. Copies Each Issue During Preceding 12 Months	No. Copies of Single Issue Published Nearest to Filing Date
a. Total Number of Copies (Net press run)			128	155
b. Paid Circulation (By Mail and Outside the Mail)	(1)	Mailed Outside-County Paid Subscriptions Stated on PS Form 3541 (Include paid distribution above nominal rate, advertiser's proof copies, and exchange copies)	64	92
	(2)	Mailed In-County Paid Subscriptions Stated on PS Form 3541 (Include paid distribution above nominal rate, advertiser's proof copies, and exchange copies)	0	0
	(3)	Paid Distribution Outside the Mails Including Sales Through Dealers and Carriers, Street Vendors, Counter Sales, and Other Paid Distribution Outside USPS®	20	30
	(4)	Paid Distribution by Other Classes of Mail Through the USPS (e.g., First-Class Mail®)	0	0
c. Total Paid Distribution (Sum of 15b (1), (2), (3), and (4))		▸	84	122
d. Free or Nominal Rate Distribution (By Mail and Outside the Mail)	(1)	Free or Nominal Rate Outside-County Copies included on PS Form 3541	34	19
	(2)	Free or Nominal Rate In-County Copies Included on PS Form 3541	0	0
	(3)	Free or Nominal Rate Copies Mailed at Other Classes Through the USPS (e.g., First-Class Mail)	0	0
	(4)	Free or Nominal Rate Distribution Outside the Mail (Carriers or other means)	0	0
e. Total Free or Nominal Rate Distribution (Sum of 15d (1), (2), (3) and (4))		▸	34	19
f. Total Distribution (Sum of 15c and 15e)		▸	118	141
g. Copies not Distributed (See Instructions to Publishers #4 (page #3))		▸	10	14
h. Total (Sum of 15f and g)		▸	128	155
i. Percent Paid (15c divided by 15f times 100)			71.19%	86.52%

* If you are claiming electronic copies, go to line 16 on page 3. If you are not claiming electronic copies, skip to line 17 on page 3.

16. Electronic Copy Circulation		Average No. Copies Each Issue During Preceding 12 Months	No. Copies of Single Issue Published Nearest to Filing Date
a. Paid Electronic Copies	▸		
b. Total Paid Print Copies (Line 15c) + Paid Electronic Copies (Line 16a)	▸		
c. Total Print Distribution (Line 15f) + Paid Electronic Copies (Line 16a)	▸		
d. Percent Paid (Both Print & Electronic Copies) (16b divided by 16c × 100)	▸		

☒ I certify that 50% of all my distributed copies (electronic and print) are paid above a nominal price.

17. Publication of Statement of Ownership

☒ If the publication is a general publication, publication of this statement is required. Will be printed in the NOVEMBER 2019 issue of this publication. ☐ Publication not required.

18. Signature and Title of Editor, Publisher, Business Manager, or Owner

STEPHEN R. BUSHING - INVENTORY DISTRIBUTION CONTROL MANAGER

Date 9/18/2019

I certify that all information furnished on this form is true and complete. I understand that anyone who furnishes false or misleading information on this form or who omits material or information requested on the form may be subject to criminal sanctions (including fines and imprisonment) and/or civil sanctions (including civil penalties).

PS Form **3526**, July 2014 (Page 3 of 4) PRIVACY NOTICE: See our privacy policy on www.usps.com

Moving?

Make sure your subscription moves with you!

To notify us of your new address, find your **Clinics Account Number** (located on your mailing label above your name), and contact customer service at:

Email: journalscustomerservice-usa@elsevier.com

800-654-2452 (subscribers in the U.S. & Canada)
314-447-8871 (subscribers outside of the U.S. & Canada)

Fax number: 314-447-8029

Elsevier Health Sciences Division
Subscription Customer Service
3251 Riverport Lane
Maryland Heights, MO 63043

*To ensure uninterrupted delivery of your subscription, please notify us at least 4 weeks in advance of move.